The Author

Audrey Eyton is the woman who can justly claim to have invented that now popular feature of every magazine stall – the slimming magazine. When she and her partner founded *Slimming Magazine* twelve years ago it was the first publication in the world to specialize in the subject. The magazine was started as a 'cottage industry', on practically no capital, because no one else believed there was enough to write on the subject, regularly. How wrong they were! The magazine was an instant success and has continued to be the dominating bestseller despite the many rival publications which have followed.

For many years Audrey Eyton edited the magazine herself, and later became Editorial Director. During their years of ownership (the company was sold in 1980) she and her partner also started Ragdale Hall Health Farm and founded and developed one of Britain's largest chains of slimming clubs. Mrs Eyton continues to work as a consultant to the company.

During her many years of specialization in this subject, Mrs Eyton has worked with most of the world's leading nutritional, medical and psychological experts. No writer has a greater knowledge and understanding of the subject. She has become an expert in her own right.

She has a fifteen-year-old son, and lives in Kensington and Kent.

Audrey Eyton

The F-Plan Diet

Combined with

The F-Plan Calorie and Fibre Charts

Charts compiled and recipes devised by
Joyce Hughes, B.Sc.
Research directed by Dr. Elizabeth Evans

The F-Plan
First serialized in the Daily Express
Published in Penguin Books 1982
Published by Allen Lane 1982

The F-Plan Calorie and Fibre Chart
Published in Penguin Books 1982

This edition first published in Great Britain in 1983 by
Octopus Books Limited
in collaboration with
Penguin Books Limited

Published in 1987 by
Treasure Press
59 Grosvenor St
London W1

ISBN 1 85051 185 3

Printed in Czechoslovakia

50648/1

Contents

As with all slimming diets, if you suffer from any health problems at all, or intend to follow a strict regime of less than 1,000 calories, check with your doctor before embarking on a dieting programme.

Acknowledgements

In addition to my excellent collaborators, Joyce Hughes and Elizabeth Evans, I would like to express my warmest gratitude to Dr David Southgate of the Food Research Institute, to Derek Miller of London University's Department of Nutrition and to Dr Martin Eastwood of the Western General Hospital, Edinburgh, all of whom have been most generous with their help and encouragement. My thanks, too, to Sue Horsman, without whose supersonic typing I would never reach a deadline, to my research assistant, Simon Sharples B.A., and to my son Matthew who, even when I delve into the sombre depths of the lower intestine, can always be relied on to come up with the jokes.

Preface

In the early spring of 1982, Linda Cook, one of the volunteers who had agreed to test a highly unusual new slimming diet, revisited London University's Department of Nutrition for her first week's weight check. Linda, Matron of the Royal Leamington Spa Nursing Home, hadn't told her own staff that she was on a diet because ... well, frankly, she had great doubts about whether she was losing any weight on it.

She had been eating meals like baked beans on toast and foods like baked potatoes. That was what – to her great surprise – she had been told to eat and she had followed instructions precisely. But after years of being indoctrinated, along with the rest of the British public, with the idea that such foods were 'fattening' she retained some of her doubts.

An even greater cause of doubt about her weight loss was the fact that she didn't feel at all hungry. Previous dieting regimes had always been accompanied by that 'half empty' feeling which this time was strangely lacking. She found it hard to imagine that she could be shedding weight without it. So it was with little optimism that she stepped on the scales to be weighed by Dr Elizabeth Evans, who was supervising the diet trials at the University.

Linda had lost 8lb in her first week on the F-Plan.

The following week she shed a further 5lb.

By the end of the third week she was as lean as a greyhound, having shed every one of her 17 surplus pounds of weight.

Linda, along with many other F-Plan dieters on the University's test panel, had shed surplus weight considerably more quickly than ever before, and with an ease which she declared to be 'absolutely staggering'. Her experience, later to be shared by hundreds of thousands of other Britons, demonstrates the F-Plan phenomenon.

The F-Plan diet has literally swept the country. At no time in history have so many Britons been shedding weight on the same diet. During the early weeks, despite herculean efforts by printer and publisher, it was nearly impossible to get *The F-Plan* into the bookshops as speedily as it was being snapped up and borne off by an eager public. The book rapidly became the fastest-selling book in the almost fifty years history of Penguin Books, selling twice as quickly as the previous record-holder, *Lady Chatterley's Lover*, when her ladyship came off the banned list in the 1960s amid an unprecedented tumult of publicity.

The F-Plan and *The F-Plan Calorie and Fibre Chart* have consistently headed Britain's bestseller lists since they were first published. The sensation created has made front-page news in the *Sunday Times*. *The F-Plan* has already sold, in a matter of months, hundreds of thousands more copies than all the American bestsellers put together – Atkins, Scarsdale, Pritikin, Mazel – have sold collectively in Britain over a period of many years.

Along with the Falklands crisis and the royal baby, The F-Plan was Britain's major talking topic of 1982. It became the subject of a Giles cartoon in the *Daily Express* and of Miles Kington's popular column in *The Times*; it featured in dozens of radio and television programmes and even in the mid-morning banter of Wogan and Young on Radio 2.

The F-Plan has caused 'happenings' that have never been known before in Britain. A near-famine of bran hit the country. Baked beans bounced off the supermarket shelves at such a rate that a puzzled supermarket manager in Bristol phoned the manufacturers to discover 'what on earth was happening'. Shops all over the country painted their windows with the slogan, 'F-Plan ingredients sold here'. A restaurant in Newcastle added F-Plan sandwiches for dieters to its lunch-time menu. So did a works canteen in Middlesex, and found that so many of the staff were following the diet that this became the top-selling lunch.

The F-Plan appeal is universal. TV stations decided to feature it because so many of their own staff were following the diet. Woman's page editors of newspapers reported on their own weight loss, and the SDP's Dr David Owen proudly announced his personal F-Plan weight loss of a stone in three weeks.

A duchess was spotted carrying the book and buying in her supplies at the local shop; whole villages and entire offices got together to shed their surplus pounds. A keen-eyed journalist in Scotland sighted a copy on the desk of the portly Lord Provost. And – the author's own favourite story – a company director from Kent phoned to tell her that the vicar, on his regular call, had refused biscuits with his tea because he was on the F-Plan.

Why all the fuss? Why such a sensation? And how was it that a diet-weary public has appreciated, with such perception and alacrity, that the F-Plan is not just another diet, but the start of a complete revolution that has upturned decades of outdated theories on dieting and that will influence slimming methods for decades to come?

The *Daily Express*, swift to spot the significance of the F-Plan, first introduced it to their readers and thus tempted many Britons to give this diet a try. But what happened after that – the enormous build-up of enthusiasm and interest – was a simple multiplication of the Linda Cook story, many thousands of times.

People tried the F-Plan, found they could keep to it, discovered they were losing weight more easily and speedily than ever before, and triumphantly told their friends: 'It works!' And thus the news spread.

The real reason for the F-Plan sensation is summed up in those two words. It works.

Introduction

Over the past years, many claims have been made suggesting that the inclusion of some particular food in a slimming diet would specifically help overweight people to shed weight more quickly and effectively. Grapefruit was a classic example. Grapefruit diets were popular for years. More recently, in an American bestseller, pineapple was invested with those magical weight-shedding properties. Sadly, *all* these claims in the past were based on fiction rather than fact – certainly not on any established medical fact! Apart from caffeine (which does have a small effect in speeding up the metabolism) no substance we eat or drink was proved by scientific methods to have any realistic effect in speeding away our surplus fat. Weight loss depended entirely on the calories we *didn't* eat.

Now, for the first time in the history of medical science, a substance has been isolated about which it is possible to say: 'If you base your slimming diet on this food you should shed weight more quickly and easily than on a diet based on the same quantity of any other foods.'

The substance is dietary fibre. This is what the F-Plan is all about. The F-Plan shows you how to cut your calorie intake and at the same time increase your intake of dietary fibre from the unrefined cereal foods and the fruits and vegetables which provide it.

When you follow the F-Plan you should:

1. Find slimming easier than ever before, because your diet will be considerably more satisfying and filling than any diet you have ever followed;

2. Lose weight *more quickly* than ever before, because a larger proportion of the calories you consume will remain undigested;

3. Gain all the well-established health advantages of eating meals high in dietary fibre content.

Who says so?

Not some earnest, eager and ignorant lady running a slimming clinic in Slough. Not some dubious doctor (all professions have their black sheep!) cashing in on some personal theory totally unsupported by scientific evidence. Who – or rather *what* – says so is a very large and growing body of evidence produced from medical research conducted by leading doctors and scientists of the Western world: experts whose reputation is beyond question and who have no cash benefit to gain from their findings.

This is what makes the F-Plan unique.

Quote: '*It seems likely that a diet in which sugars and starches are taken in natural fibre-rich form would contribute to the control of obesity by encouraging satiety at a lower level of energy intake, and to a lesser extent by increasing the amount of potential energy lost in the faeces.*'

What that means, in simple English, is that if you follow a high-fibre diet you will find that you feel more satisfied on fewer calories. And more of the calories that go into your mouth will, to put it bluntly, go straight through and down the lavatory.

Of course, the fewer calories the body uses from food the more it must draw from your surplus body fat, so this adds up to faster weight loss.

Another simple definition which will appeal to everyone who has ever tried to slim: More weight loss for less willpower!

Even more dramatic: *who* made the statement quoted above? The answer is that august, eminent and necessarily highly conservative body, the Royal College of Physicians. This statement is drawn from the special report they have compiled on the medical aspects of dietary fibre. The members of the Royal College need a very large quantity of scientific evidence indeed, drawn from many sources, before they will commit themselves so far. If they feel it likely that a high-fibre diet, which also reduces sugar and fat, will be particularly beneficial to slimmers – as they do – we need hardly say more. The F-Plan is the first slimming diet which enables you to follow this formula.

These discoveries are recent for a particular reason: medical scientists only started seriously investigating the benefits of high-fibre diets ten years ago. Before that time, only a minority of 'cranks' insisted on eating wholemeal bread, extolling the virtues of bran, and complaining of the ill-effects of a Western diet rich in refined carbo-hydrates.

When the authentic medical researchers started to get involved, they were looking for dietary answers to serious illnesses prevalent in West-ern societies but extremely rare in many less sophisticated communities in the developing world. Why was it that so many diseases, like cancer and other disorders of the bowel, heart disease and diabetes, were occurring frequently here, but not there? What were these people doing that we weren't doing, and vice versa? One of the answers which emerged was that they were eating diets high in natural fibre – while we, in the West, were stripping this cell-wall material from our day-to-day diet by refining our cereal foods and sugar.

In recent years the evidence for the health benefits of fibre, or 'roughage' as it used to be called, has grown so strong that it has filtered through from the medical journals and is now well known to the British and American public. These days it isn't just those health-food cranks who are scurrying off to buy their brown wholemeal loaves. Sales of this typical high-fibre food are measurably increasing all the time. The health connection was the motivation for the research that led to keen medical interest and the endorsement of the benefits of dietary fibre. The slimming connection has emerged more recently, almost as an accidental byproduct of this research.

In addition to being relatively free from many major diseases, those people in developing countries, eating their high-fibre diets, were found to escape another major scourge of Western civilization – obesity. Even where food is plentiful, societies accustomed to a diet containing a high percentage of cereal foods, fruit and vegetables, all rich in natural fibre, do not become overweight.

This intriguing finding from the surveys led medical researchers to investigations into a whole new aspect of dietary fibre. Why were those high-fibre eaters keeping slim even when they were eating their fill? Could it be that the calories supplied by a diet high in natural fibre were being digested and utilized in a different way by the human body? The remarkable answer, revealed by many recent scientific experiments, is undoubtedly: YES.

However, today's enlightened experts realize that there is little point in discovering important diet guidelines unless these can be presented to the public in a form which makes them realistic and easy to incorporate into daily eating.

On this principle, Dr Elizabeth Evans has worked most diligently in supervising research, and Derek Miller, the distinguished nutritional expert, has made research information and facilities available to us at London University. At the Food Research Institute Dr David Southgate, who has made a special study of dietary fibre and whose research is the source of the scientific textbook fibre figures, has provided analytical values for the dietary fibre in a range of usefully fibre-rich canned and packaged foods, so that for the first time these products, which form such a major part of modern eating, can be realistically assessed and used for health value.

Another expert in the work on dietary fibre, Dr Martin Eastwood of Edinburgh's Western General Hospital, has generously given his advice and guidance, and Joyce Hughes, who lectures in nutrition at Croydon College, has compiled the F-Plan calorie and fibre charts.

There can be no doubt about the authenticity of the F-Plan and its claim that dietary fibre will help you slim. But on the basis that 'there has to be a snag', those who haven't taken much interest in the dietary fibre health factor to date may well become a little alarmed about what type of foods they will be required to eat on this diet. Somehow the words 'dietary fibre' do tend to conjure up an image of being put out to graze on food that has all the comfort and flavour of that consumed by a sheep or a cow.

When we tell you that baked beans on toast (as long as the toast is made with wholemeal bread) is one of the best high-fibre meals you can eat, it should give great reassurance to those who enjoy the more homely delights of the table. A quick glance at the recipes in the second part of this book should delight the gastronomically adventurous.

Dietary fibre is provided by a wide selection of easily available and palatable foods. The F-Plan will provide you with a wonderfully easy formula for boosting your intake to between 35g and 50g of fibre a day – at least twice most people's normal consumption – without sacrificing any pleasure in meals.

Those readers who are now sufficiently convinced that the F-Plan is the first realistically helpful medical advance in slimming, as indeed it is, may if they wish turn to page 91 of this book, where they will find all the rules for following the plan, followed by recipes, menus and charts.

The F-Plan calorie and fibre charts are the first charts to make it possible to keep to the correct number of calories and, at the same time, to choose the foods which will be of most help in making slimming both easier and speedier. For the health-conscious person, as well as those concerned about weight, they are a unique guide, making it possible to follow that major modern nutritional recommendation made by all leading medical authorities in the Western world: increase your intake of dietary fibre.

You will find three food charts in this book (in addition to a calorie chart of drinks) to make it triply easy to follow the new high-fibre low-calorie method of eating reduction and health benefit.

The first makes it easy to see which foods are low in calories and which are high in dietary fibre by listing the calorie and fibre content of average or easily recognizable portions of all the basic foods. You will see at a glance the number of calories and the quantity of dietary fibre (when present) in a whole average-sized eating apple, or a carrot, or a rasher of bacon. We call this chart the 'Instant Calorie and Fibre Guide'.

Our next chart, the 'Calorie and Fibre Guide to Packaged Foods', makes high-fibre low-calorie eating even easier. In this we reveal the number of calories and the quantity of dietary fibre present in the useful canned and packaged foods. The use of convenience foods need be no crime in health and weight control if the correct ones are chosen: in fact they can be a great asset. Here is the guide you need.

'Your Basic Calorie and Fibre Chart', reveals the calorie and fibre content (where present) of all those basic everyday foods on a per ounce basis.

However, we hope that you will take time to read the chapters that precede the recipes, menus and diet charts. Because if you do, you cannot fail to be deeply impressed by the very many ways in which high-fibre foods can help you to slim, and to come to the conclusion that the F-Plan is that major slimming breakthrough everyone has been seeking for so long.

I

What (and where) is dietary fibre?

Dietary fibre is a substance obtained from plant foods, as distinct from animal foods. All cereals, fruits and vegetables contain some dietary fibre, but, just as the calorie content of different foods varies to a great degree, so does the fibre content of different plant foods. Some are excellent sources, while the quantity contained in an average serving of others would be negligible. With cereal-based foods, fibre value depends to a large degree on how much has been stripped away in the milling and refining processes. Fruits and vegetables, even in their raw, unprocessed state, differ so much that you certainly can't say that *all* of them are useful sources of fibre.

But precisely what is dietary fibre? Well, it could be loosely defined as the cell-wall material of plants – but only loosely, because it also consists of substances associated with these cell walls. Dietary fibre can also be described as the carbohydrate material in plant foods (mainly derived from the cell walls) which is not digested by man. Note that phrase 'not digested by man', because it gives you your first clue to the slimming advantages of dietary fibre. Food which is not digested cannot be used to provide body fat or calories!

All plants and animals, ourselves included, are made up of cells, but the cell walls of plants are of a more rigid structure. This performs the function of enclosing cell contents, trapping water, stiffening the plant and conducting sap. It is tempting to think of dietary fibre as the tough stuff which holds the plant together, and this is true to a degree, but it can be misleading when it comes to locating high-fibre plants by guesswork. Cell walls are made up of a variety of substances of which only one, cellulose, is truly fibrous in the sense of being filamentous or threadlike.

Hence if you were to take a guess at selecting a high-fibre vegetable you might well think of something like celery, which seems to reveal its fibre content unmistakably. Yet peas, extolled by advertisers for their tenderness, in fact contain more than four times the fibre of celery, weight for weight.

Generally, however, high-fibre foods do require more chewing, which gives them yet another slimming advantage, as you will learn later in this book.

Unless you have been living on another planet for the past few years, you will be under the impression that bran is high in dietary fibre and you will be absolutely correct. It consists largely of cell-wall material from grain and contains between 40 and 50 per cent dietary fibre – a much greater percentage than any other food. Bran is a byproduct of the milling process used in making white and other extracted flours. It is largely because the bran is stripped from white flour and, similarly, because the cell-wall material is stripped from sugar cane and sugar beet, that our Western diet has become low in natural fibre content. White flour, the basis of so many foods, is fibre-depleted flour. Sugar, as we use it, is sugar cane or beet totally divested of all its dietary fibre.

However, the F-Plan does not require you to obtain your dietary fibre from bran alone. Yesterday's message of 'bran alone' is now outdated and for some very good reasons. For one thing, bran is a bulky substance and it isn't easy to consume much more than half an ounce a day without making your diet unpalatable.

So although we all know that bran is the richest of all sources of dietary fibre, in the percentage it contains, if you have tried sprinkling it on breakfast cereal and weighed the quantity, you will have discovered that you get a large volume in a quarter of an ounce. Just about as much as you can palatably add to a single portion of breakfast cereal, without beginning to think that you are eating a bowl of sawdust.

Most people would only eat bran with breakfast cereal. Yes, there are enthusiasts who scatter it on to their scallops, mash it into their spinach and, quite possibly, stir it into their tea. But in the F-Plan we use bran only where it is palatable. No one ever goes on eating anything they don't like for long.

More important, though, is the fact that dietary fibre differs in some degree from plant to plant. It is a complex substance and there is still much to be learned about it. Medical researchers are becoming increasingly aware of the health and weight-control benefits of dietary fibre in general – but the indications are that different forms of fibre may perform different beneficial functions.

Fresh fruit, for instance, being mainly water, provides only a dilute

form of dietary fibre. Weight for weight it does not compare favour-
ably with foods like cereals and nuts in fibre content, although it
works out well when you take into account how much fibre you get for
a modest number of calories. However, there is a substance called
pectin, which is part of the fibre of fruit, which is not found in other
plant foods. Medical experiments indicate that the presence of an
appreciable quantity of pectin in the diet tends to increase the number
of calories excreted in the stools in the form of fat. Obviously, the
more calories you excrete the more calories the body is deprived of,
and the more speedily you force it to shed weight.

For this and other known and yet to be investigated reasons, it is
obviously a good plan to boost daily fibre intake – for health and
slimming benefit – from a variety of cereal, fruit and vegetable sources,
and this is what you do on the F-Plan. Although the benefits of
dietary fibre are still in the process of scientific investigation, we want
to make sure that you don't miss out on any of the advantages, both
those which are known and those still to be fully revealed.

Although generally aware that bran, wholemeal bread (which has
less of its fibre stripped away in the milling process than white bread)
and muesli-type mixtures are rich sources of fibre, most people find it.
difficult to know where to locate that healthy high-fibre food. There
is a good reason for this difficulty. So far, no one seems to have
compiled a really helpful and realistic guide to the sources of fibre in
everyday foods. It is possible to consult scientific textbooks and discover the percentage of fibre in various cereal foods, fruits and vegetables. But this is only part of the story and can be very misleading.

To assess realistically how much fibre a particular food is likely to
contribute to a daily menu, it is important to estimate what quantity of
that particular food you are likely to eat. This varies a great deal from
food to food.

Let us consider watercress as a typical example of how easy it is to
be deceived. If you were to consult fibre charts, you would see that
watercress (3·3 per cent fibre) appears to be quite a good source. It
contains a higher percentage of fibre than cabbage, for instance, and
more than twice as much as apples on a weight-for-weight basis.
However, if you were to help yourself to a reasonably generous helping
of watercress as part of a salad meal, it is unlikely that your portion
would weigh more than half an ounce. You get plenty of watercress

for half an ounce, but the quantity of dietary fibre in that weight is really too small to make any realistic contribution to your daily intake. It provides you with just half a gram of fibre. If you were to serve yourself an average helping of cabbage, though, it would usually weigh at least two ounces if you were eating it raw as part of a portion of coleslaw, for example, or four ounces if you were serving boiled cabbage. If you were to pick up and weigh that apple you are about to eat, you would find it weighed about five ounces. So both these foods are useful sources of dietary fibre because, unlike watercress, they tend to be consumed in reasonably weighty quantities. The apple would provide more than two grams of fibre, and the cooked cabbage nearly three.

Why we eat what we do and how much we eat of any particular food is a fascinating subject. It depends a good deal on the bulk and 'fillability' of the food, of course. Hence many of the fibre-rich foods have inbuilt quantity controls because of their sheer bulk – fruit and vegetables in particular.

But there are many other factors involved. We tend to serve and finish off complete units of food as provided for us by manufacturers. If you are wondering, for instance, why The Instant Calorie and Fibre Chart lists only three quarters of an ounce of shredded wheat and then an ounce or more of other cereals, ask yourself whether you have ever seen anyone eat one and a quarter, or perhaps one and one third, shredded wheats . . . There are those who eat one shredded wheat and those who eat two. The world is precisely divided between those two groups with no grey areas in between.

Similarly, with potato crisps, have you ever known anyone *not* finish a packet they started? There are even some (not you, of course!) who have been known to lick the first finger of the right hand and dip it into the bottom of the packet, so that those tiny remaining crumbs of crisp can be finished off.

Nature does a neat packaging job with many foods, of course, and this also influences the quantity we normally consume. Where one unit is usually sufficient to satisfy the appetite and desire, we tend to keep to just one unit – one apple, one pear, one orange. Where mother nature has been meaner in her packaged quantity, with plums for instance, one unit does not have an inbuilt stop mechanism, so we often end up eating a good deal more than we would with a larger fruit. This has been taken into account in compiling The Instant Calorie and Fibre Chart, too.

How we buy food also has an influence on how much we eat of it at any one meal. If we buy half a pound we tend to eat either half a pound – or half that quantity.

The size of the dish or plate we use affects quantity as well, and this mainly accounts for the variation in quantities of breakfast cereals. Where a cereal is very light, like cornflakes, an ounce will comfortably fill the usual breakfast bowl. With Puffed Wheat an ounce would actually overflow in many bowls, so people tend to serve less than an ounce. Bran cereals and muesli are rather more weighty, so here people tend to serve out more than an ounce just so that it looks sufficient.

Price is another factor which influences quantity with some foods – mainly those we think of as protein foods. For example, most people will be quite content with a two-ounce portion of prawns, because they have become accustomed to eating a modest quantity of an expensive food, while with many fish – cod, for instance – six ounces would be a more usual serving. This factor applies less with foods rich in dietary fibre, because these foods – happily – tend to be inexpensive. But it might influence the quantities of grapes or strawberries consumed, for instance.

The amount of work we have to do in consuming any particular food influences the quantity too – both chewing (where high-fibre foods score so well) and manual work. Scientists discovered, in an experiment with overweight people, that when allowed to eat as much as they wanted, they ate considerably fewer peanuts in the shell than peanuts provided ready-shelled.

On the whole, the bulky form of foods rich in dietary fibre has a wonderful restraining effect on the quantity consumed – one of the great advantages of the F-Plan. But use self-control in relation to nuts (it's a good idea to buy them in shells) and take care with dried fruit – we have observed that some slimmers make frequent sorties into the pantry to nibble a handful of dried fruit. This way rather a lot of calories can be consumed; the chart gives the number of calories per ounce of dried fruit.

Dried fruit has been processed, of course, to some degree. It is interesting to note how often foods only become fattening when man has had a hand in processing them in some way. The foods which are consumed very much in the way they were grown – many of the fibre-rich foods – are rarely potentially fattening. It would appear that God did not intend us to be fat.

The best sources of all are those foods which have a high percentage of fibre and tend also to be consumed in reasonably large quantities . . . without providing too many calories, if you are slimming! This is where, for instance, the good old baked bean in tomato sauce is unbeatable. These beans consist of more than seven per cent dietary fibre and most people would eat the contents of an 8oz can. This means that an average serving would contribute more than 16g of fibre to the diet, which is more than half the quantity that the average Briton consumes in a day on his fibre-depleted diet.

At the other end of the scale, one of the poorer vegetable sources of fibre is cucumber, which contains only 0·4 per cent of dietary fibre and tends to be consumed in modest servings. It has a low fibre content and a low portion weight, so its fibre contribution to the average diet is negligible.

Taking this essential 'how much is normally eaten' factor into account we have compiled the guide starting on page 213. This gives a truly realistic and helpful guide to the fibre content of foods. Based on average portions, it shows you a whole range of foods, from those which are enormously helpful to those which are virtually useless in boosting the fibre content of your diet.

2

The vital calorie factor

By including sufficient high-fibre foods in your diet you will actually help your body to shed surplus fat. But this doesn't mean that you can forget about calories. The strength of the F-Plan lies in the way it affects the calories you consume.

Never let anyone, or any diet, convince you that calories don't count in achieving weight loss. They do. They are what slimming is all about.

Calories are units of energy, the energy we need to keep going. We consume these calories in the form of food and use them up in maintaining the body's functions and movements. All foods supply calories, but in widely varying quantities on an ounce-for-ounce basis.

Sometimes – often, in fact – in the Western world, people consume more calories than they need to fuel the body with energy. A percentage of these surplus calories is then stored as body fat, and this is what makes people overweight.

The only way in which to reverse this situation and become slim again is to supply the body with fewer calories than it needs for its daily energy requirements, so that it has to draw on the emergency store of calories in its own fat. When you are slimming you are really eating your own body – eating away the part of it you don't want, that surplus fat! Apart from becoming highly energetic and making the body burn up many more calories daily – a possible but usually very slow method of shedding weight – there is no other way of losing weight than by depriving the body of calories.

All slimming diets which can possibly work are based on calorie reduction, but it is easy to see why people become confused about this. So many diets appear to have no connection with calories.

An example is the once highly popular low-carbohydrate method of slimming. Dieters were told that they only had to ration carbohydrates and then they could eat as much as they liked of other foods. These diets are now frowned upon by many medical experts because of their low fibre content. However, it is true that many people have succeeded in shedding weight on them in the past. (These diets could be said to have been half-right, in that they did cut out refined carbohydrates, but unfortunately without adding fibre-rich carbohydrate foods which we now know to be of such help to slimmers.)

The reason for weight loss, though, was calorie reduction. Because so many people in the West eat such a large proportion of their daily calories in the form of refined sugary and starchy foods, it was found that, when these foods were strictly rationed, daily calorie intake usually automatically dropped sufficiently to achieve weight loss. Although people were allowed to eat other foods freely, in fact when they were deprived of their refined carbohydrates they tended not to increase their intake of these alternative foods very much – not enough to make up for the calories they were saving.

Then there are those modern diets which tell you to ration only fats. Fats supply the most calories of all, very many more, weight for weight, than all other foods. All high-calorie foods are fatty, and all high calorie meals are fatty. So by rationing these foods you cut calorie intake. You are on a low-calorie diet. But since the foods allowed are still refined foods, the fibre content may not be high enough to meet present recommended levels.

Ah, but what about this remarkable new diet formula from America which tells you that you can eat vast quantities of melon and chicken, or spinach and prunes, or pineapple, or whatever, as long as you keep to this one food, or this combination of two foods, for the whole day? You may have actually heard people raving about the miracle weight losses they have achieved and attributed to these magical foods. Poor souls, all they were doing was cutting calorie intake – the hard way. You could say their success was based on the 'throw-up factor'. There is a limit to the quantity of any one particular food you can eat, and continue to eat without other foods, before beginning to feel bored with it and then almost sick at the thought of it.

More scientifically, variety has been found to be a factor in influencing the quantity of food we desire. It is partly because our Western diets are varied (and healthily so, because this ensures a wide range of necessary vitamins and minerals) that we are tempted to overeat. It's amazing how easy and tempting it is to eat a little more when we are offered food of a different flavour and texture – the dessert after a savoury meal, for instance. Interestingly enough, even hens and rats have been found to consume more calories when they are offered a varied diet than when they are fed 'the same old thing' all the time.

People eating 'the same old thing' eat fewer calories. Restrict a person to any one food and – even if that food is chocolate – they will almost certainly shed weight. But these diets are, by their nature, eventually self-defeating. After a certain time the very sight of the food allowed becomes off-putting and even repellent. Many people have experience of this from gorging sessions in childhood. My own son, as a small boy, allowed to graze freely on a strawberry field during a 'pick your own' expedition and aware that he, unlike our basket, would not be weighed and charged, once achieved a mammoth strawberry-eating feat. That was five years ago, and he hasn't been able to face a strawberry since!

So ALL diets, even those which come complete with generally useless injections and pills, achieve weight loss only by reducing calorie intake.

The F-Plan also reduces your calorie intake in order to allow you to shed weight at sufficient speed. But the radical difference between this and previous dieting methods is that it makes the food you consume more filling and also renders some of the calories it supplies non-fattening, as you will begin to learn in the next chapter.

3

The calorie–fibre connection

The most dramatic thing about the recent dietary fibre research is that it has, to a degree, altered the basis on which experts have been calculating potential weight loss over the past half century or so ... the period during which overweight people have been begging diet doctors and dieticians to help them shed that surplus fat.

It is never possible to predict weight loss precisely. Even on the same diet, this will vary from person to person depending on many individual factors, including the amount of excess weight (the heavier you are the faster you tend to shed weight) and the degree of energy expended in physical activity. Nevertheless, there was a simple weight-loss equation on which it was possible to estimate the maximum amount of weight likely to be lost each week on any specific calorie allowance. This was based on subtracting the calories consumed in food from the calories required to keep the body going.

Let us assume that you are a woman of medium height, doing a job like housework, which requires a moderate amount of physical activity, and that you are about one stone overweight and just about to embark on trying to lose it. In these circumstances, it could be roughly assumed that you would be burning up around 2,000 calories a day.

If we were to put you on a slimming diet providing you with 1,500 calories a day, you would be 500 calories short of your requirement and these would have to be taken from your body fat. It has been scientifically estimated that a pound of your own body fat provides approximately 3,500 calories. So during a week you would be likely to shed one pound of surplus fat.

Obviously, if you followed a stricter diet, allowing you only 1,000 calories a day, you would draw an additional 500 calories a day from your body fat. So with a daily deficit of 1,000 calories you could expect to shed around two pounds a week.

As you see, expected rate of fat loss has always been estimated simply by counting the calories consumed in the form of food, any food, and subtracting them from the number the body requires for energy.

The recent findings about fibre introduce a new factor into this weight-loss equation.

As you read in the introduction to this book, when people eat high-fibre diets they excrete more calories in their stools (faeces). In several experiments, scientists have undertaken the task of analysing the stools of those following high-fibre diets and have found that the calories excreted are measurably greater in number than the calories excreted by those on the normal, varied Western diets, rich in refined carbohydrate foods – or, indeed, on any other pattern of eating. Tests indicate that the increased calorie content of the faeces amounts to nearly ten per cent when people follow high-fibre diets.

Obviously, those calories which are being flushed away are not being used by the body . . . which means that the body is having to use more of its own surplus fat to make up for them. So on a 1,000 calorie high-fibre diet the body is going to shed weight more quickly than on a normal 1,000 calorie diet of varied food – or on any other 1,000 calorie diet.

Before the fascinating high-fibre research findings it was assumed that weight loss depended entirely on *the number* of calories consumed compared with the number expended by the body. Now we have to add another factor to this simple statement.

Weight loss depends on the number and the *source* of calories consumed. The rate of weight loss will be influenced not only by the quantity you eat, in terms of calories, but also by which foods you choose to make up that calorie intake.

This is a great asset in favour of high-fibre dieting, but is very far from being the only advantage you gain when you follow the F-Plan slimming method. The benefit of this revolutionary diet is based not on just one advantage over other diets but on many factors which add up to faster, easier, more effective slimming. The fact is that from the moment you put fibre-rich food into your mouth it starts to give both physical and psychological advantages in filling you, satisfying you, protecting you from feeling hungry again soon, and speeding your weight loss.

The slimming benefits of the F-Plan diet start in the mouth, continue in the stomach, extend to the blood and reach a grand finale with that final flush!

So let's start with the first mouthful and work our way down the whole digestive tract, to explain fully the marvellous benefits of this new slimming method.

4

How fibre helps – in your mouth

Even before the foods which are rich in dietary fibre start to pass down your throat, they perform a multiplicity of functions which help to reduce the quantity of food you want to eat and they start to send helpful satiety signals to the brain. A whole range of slimming benefits, both physiological and psychological, come into play right there in your mouth.

One of these benefits is in slowing down your eating. This may not, at first glance, seem to be a major factor but in fact it is a crucial element in weight control. The rate at which you eat not only strongly influences how much you want to eat but – more surprisingly – it influences the length of time elapsing before you feel the desire to eat again. One of the most fascinating scientific experiments of recent years showed that when people ate meals at a rapid rate they became hungry again more quickly than when they ate precisely the same size of meal at a slower rate. Why this happens isn't fully understood. But it is well endorsed by general observation.

Never underestimate the role of eating-speed in slimming and weight control. It is very much more important than most people realize. If a group of people sitting at a dining table had their entire bodies shrouded under some tent-like garment, there are two ways in which the expert observer of eating behaviour could differentiate the fat from the slim. One of the things the expert would note would be that, however big the meal – and let us assume that over-large portions were served – some people would consume every morsel and leave an entirely clean plate. These would almost certainly be the overweight people, and this is something you can observe for yourself in almost any restaurant.

Overweight people, particularly the heavily overweight, rarely stop eating until they have finished everything on the plate. Slim people, in contrast, usually stop when they feel satisfied. In the case of an over-large meal this would mean that the slim people would put down their knives and forks and leave some food.

Overweight people seem to lack a 'stop mechanism'. This appears to be one of their basic problems. Effortlessly slim people are governed by their body's requirement for food and are bullied by messages from the body — 'That's it, old chap, I've had enough' — at the appropriate time. 'Honestly,' they say, 'I couldn't eat another morsel.' And they really mean it.

In contrast, overweight people seem to get much less strong and effective stop signals from the body, and this is largely because of the other factor, the major clue, which our eating-behaviour expert would be using in his 'guess who's overweight' game.

The overweight people would eat more rapidly than the slim people. This has been shown in several scientific experiments which invariably indicate that overweight people eat more quickly than slim people. A recent experiment in America showed that people of normal weight might start eating at a reasonably rapid pace at the beginning of a meal, when their hunger is at a peak, but this eating rate will steadily slow down as the meal progresses. The overweight people in this experiment, however, kept eating at the same fast pace throughout the meal.

Again, this is something you can observe for yourself in any public eating place. The overweight people tend to eat in a non-stop motion. As one mouthful of food is being chewed, the other is on the fork and on its way up — ready to be put in the mouth the second that the first mouthful starts on its way down the throat.

From my own observations, generally the greater the weight problem the faster the rate of eating. America, where there appear to be more grossly obese people than in Britain (by which I mean those around double their desirable body weight, rather than just a couple of stones overweight), is an excellent place to observe this eating-speed phenomenon. Once I sat with an American psychiatrist, a specialist in eating behaviour, and observed a hugely overweight couple (quite unaware that we were watching them) eating their restaurant break-fasts. The quantity of food collected from the help-yourself buffet was enormous and the speed with which it was consumed was almost supersonic. The husband not only forked food into his mouth with an almost non-stop movement of his right hand, but he also held a corn bun in his left hand so that food could be put into his mouth to fill the split second it took to reload the fork. Chewing must have been abso-lutely minimal. Needless to say, silence prevailed throughout the meal.

And at the end of it, after eating what must have been at least half-a-dozen scrambled eggs, plus bacon, sausages and several buns, the couple got up to reload their plates . . .

This is an extreme example. But most of us who have any kind of weight problem, however small, can benefit from slowing down our eating, for some very sound scientific reasons.

After food is put into the mouth it takes a few minutes (usually around five) even to start having any physical effect in satisfying the hungry body. At a fast eating pace and with a minimum amount of chewing – and very little chewing is usually required with refined sugary and starchy foods – an awful lot of calories can be consumed in five minutes.

As eating-time continues, the body sends out more and more satiety signals, but it is estimated that it takes about twenty minutes for a meal to have its full effect in filling our stomachs and sending out all the other physical signals of sufficiency. That is why speedy eaters, who eat their fill in perhaps ten or fifteen minutes, often feel over-full some minutes after the meal. Most of us, the slim as well as the overweight, have uttered that plaintive wail: 'Oh, I shouldn't have done it!', as we pat our far from comfortable stomachs after a par-ticularly tempting feast, like Christmas dinner, and stagger off for the Rennies.

'Slow down your eating' is excellent classic advice for those with a weight problem – and many of those who have struggled long in the battle of the bulge have probably read it before, and even tried to follow it. Quite probably they have failed, or given up trying after a time.

Why? Because the rate of eating is a deeply established habit and all deeply established habits are very difficult to break. If you were advised to speak more slowly it would probably take months of effort, repeated conscious effort, before you succeeded in altering the speed at which you spoke. The same would apply to changing your accent. Think of the effort that Professor Higgins had to put in with Eliza!

Slowing down a habitual eating rate isn't easy and tends to need prolonged effort. And this is where a high-fibre diet starts to play its first function in helping you to eat less. It automatically slows down the rate of eating for you! And for a number of reasons – not just one.

First of all, plant foods in their natural form, unstripped of natural fibre in processing, tend to be bulky. You get a large volume or bulk of food for a small or moderate number of calories, and that in itself is going to necessitate considerably more chewing and take considerably more time. Take sugar and apples for comparison. The average Briton consumes about five ounces of sugar in a day. In the way it is grown and gathered, in cane or beet, sugar contains an appreciable content of dietary fibre, but this is stripped away completely in the refining process to leave no fibre at all in the sugar we buy in packets or consume in cakes, biscuits or drinks.

Many people consume a good deal of sugar in drinks. It takes hardly any time at all to swoosh down a can of cola, and neither does this seem to have any effect in satisfying the appetite. Most people find it easy to drink large quantities of calorific drinks, sweet or alcoholic, without in any way lessening or delaying their appetite for the next meal – and these drinks, and sugar itself, are perhaps the ultimate example of fibre-free calories. By consuming calories without any dietary fibre at all, you can get down a very large number of calories, at a very fast rate, with very little effect in satisfying the appetite.

Even when refined sugar is combined with refined flour to make cakes or desserts, the chewing required tends to be minimal.

It is somewhat unrealistic to imagine people gnawing away at sugar cane or sugar beet, so as an example at the opposite extreme let us consider apples. Apples are basically a mixture of water, sugar, dietary fibre and little else. Only the sugar in them supplies calories. You would have to eat about a dozen apples in order to obtain that average daily 5oz of sugar from this source; you can imagine how long that would take and how difficult it would be to eat all the remainder of your daily food. If the dietary fibre were removed, the apples would become apple juice. This way, those apple sugar calories could be consumed very quickly without the appetite-satisfying effect. So it *is* the dietary fibre which has the slowing down and filling up effect.

This principle is true of all foods. Dietary fibre, which is calorie-free, has the general effect of adding bulk, slowing down eating and satisfying the appetite in this and many other ways.

But this isn't the only way in which dietary fibre slows down eating. The texture as well as the bulk of fibre-rich foods helps to put on the brakes.

The pleasure of eating is largely the pleasure of taste. In natural fibre-rich foods the taste-evoking substances appear to remain intact within the cell walls which have not been stripped away by refining processes. Therefore the taste of an unprocessed food is not fully appreciated unless it is chewed. This may be one reason why fibre-rich foods are normally automatically chewed more thoroughly than processed foods.

There is *yet another* reason why many fibre-rich foods slow down eating and add to satisfaction. Food is not swallowed with comfort unless, or until, it is soft and moist. If it is dry and unyielding we automatically chew it until it becomes comfortable to swallow. Many high-fibre fruits and vegetables, nuts and dry breakfast cereals (shredded wheat, for instance, as opposed to porridge) need a good deal of chewing before they can be comfortably swallowed. Cooking, particularly boiling, reduces but does not wholly remove the firmness of food.

Scientists have done careful experiments to confirm the benefits of dietary fibre in slowing down eating. Sensibly comparing two foods of a very similar nature, they monitored a group of people eating a 'meal' consisting entirely of wholemeal bread, which contains 8·5 per cent of dietary fibre, and compared them with a group eating a 'meal' of white bread, which contains only 2·7 per cent dietary fibre. The wholemeal bread took 11 minutes longer to consume (45 minutes) than the white bread (34 minutes).

Dietary fibre means that a food requires more chewing but it *also* requires more swallowing. During prolonged chewing, more saliva is secreted and this adds to the volume of the food in the mouth. That obviously necessitates more swallowing movements.

Although it takes a few minutes for the body to send out any strong signals of satiety it is probable that chewing and swallowing movements do begin to send messages to the brain.

All of us, the overweight as well as the slim, have some body controls which limit our eating capacity. Otherwise, some people would indeed quite literally eat themselves to death – in fact there have been a few cases of disturbed people doing just that in recent years. However, the vast majority of people have inbuilt controls and these seem to differ only in their degree of effectiveness between the overweight and the slim. The major control mechanisms appear to be the state of fullness of the stomach, the level of sugar in the blood, and a satiety centre in the brain known as the appestat.

In experiments with rats, increased electrical activity was recorded in the satiety centre of the brain during chewing and swallowing. This indicates that chewing and swallowing at least start to bring our bodily eating controls into action by sending the first satiety signals to the brain – and that the more chewing and swallowing we do the more effective this is likely to be.

So far we have dealt only with the physical benefits of fibre-rich foods in the mouth. The psychological benefits might well be just as great.

Chewing gives psychological satisfaction, and even in scientific experiments the chewing of gum has been found to help reduce tension. Psychiatrists working in the area of weight control have discovered that we need our 'psychological fill' as well as our physical fill of food in order to feel content with what we have eaten.

When someone eats a snack while mentally absorbed in other things – perhaps a mother grabbing her own meal in between attempts to coax food down a baby, or a viewer eating a T V snack while totally involved in the latest beastly plots of 'J.R.' – it has been found that the food has little effect in satisfying hunger. Often, for instance, after the baby has been put to sleep the mother will sit down and eat another meal.

We seem to need to get a sufficient daily quota of conscious relaxation and pleasure from our food, and obviously this occurs while the food is in the mouth. Little wonder that a meal of mainly refined foods, gulped down in seconds, tends to lead to second helpings to extend the time of eating, or another meal or snack shortly afterwards to 'bulk out' the eating pleasure of the day.

In this chapter you have discovered many ways in which foods containing dietary fibre can make you feel more satisfied – and the food has not yet gone down the throat. See what happens when high-fibre food reaches the stomach . . .

5

How fibre fills your stomach – and for longer

Dietary fibre is a sponge-like material which absorbs and holds water as it is chewed in the mouth and passes down the gastro-intestinal tract. This means that fibre-rich foods swell to a greater bulk, to fill the stomach, than any other foods.

The state of fullness of the stomach is obviously going to influence your appetite. A derivative of cellulose, one of the substances present in dietary fibre, has long been used as a 'slimming aid' for this reason.

Many of the pills and capsules which are sold to slimmers as appetite suppressants consist largely of methyl cellulose. The only problem is that you can't get enough of this material in pills and capsules to provide enough bulk to have any realistically helpful effect in filling the stomach.

However, when scientists Derek Miller and Dr Elizabeth Evans conducted tests at London University, adding 20g of cellulose to people's daily diet, they found this did indeed automatically reduce calorie intake. People consumed fewer calories without even trying to do so. So a sufficient quantity of cellulose does help you to eat less.

This large bulk of material in the stomach on a high-fibre diet is just one of the factors which makes you feel more satisfied on less food. Equally important is the fact that fibre-rich food *stays* in the stomach longer than fibre-depleted food. Those gastric acids have a much tougher job to do when they have to fight their way through fibrous cell-wall material. This produces two results – both beneficial in weight loss. Food in a fibre-rich diet stays in the stomach longer; and it seems probable that the food is less efficiently digested as it goes through the digestive tract.

The second factor is less obviously helpful at first glance – but what it adds up to is calorie saving!

The cell walls themselves are totally indigestible and do not provide calories. This factor is taken into account in giving the calorie values of carbohydrate foods. However, it seems highly likely that some of the calorie-supplying substances associated with the cell walls are not digested either when a diet is high in natural fibre. This would help to account for some of the extra calories expelled in the faeces of those consuming fibre-rich foods.

So when you eat your F-Plan fibre-rich diet you get a greater and more filling bulk of food in the stomach, the food stays there longer, and it is likely that fewer of those potentially fat-producing calories are digested.

Yet *another* advantage is the prevention of stomach discomfort, often the trigger for diet-breaking snacks. Unless stomach acids have a job to do in digesting food they tend to cause discomfort, and dieters often find themselves turning to extra food to quell that unpleasant acidic feeling when the stomach is largely empty. Fibre-rich foods keep the stomach acids under control for long periods because those acids have to work longer and harder at digestion processes.

It is only when the fibre-rich food leaves the stomach that it starts passing through the body at a faster pace, giving the well-documented health benefits. It stays longer where you need it to stay – in the stomach – and moves more swiftly where you need it to move more swiftly, through the intestine and bowel.

But we are far from being at the end of the chain of slimming benefits that are achieved by a diet rich in natural fibre. There is the blood factor, too, which can also provide a major benefit, as you will learn in the next chapter.

6

Rebound hunger – how fibre beats it

One of the major problems which gave carbohydrate foods in general the reputation of being fattening would be described by doctors as 'rebound hypoglycaemia'. The rest of us might put the same thing in much more simple terms by voicing that popular complaint, 'When you've eaten a Chinese meal you feel hungry again in a couple of hours.' This kind of comment might well follow a Chinese meal consisting largely of white processed rice. Carbohydrate foods – it used to be thought *all* carbohydrate foods – do indeed have a tendency to produce a rebound hunger. There is a scientific explanation.

One of the processes of digestion is to reduce food to a substance which can be absorbed in the bloodstream as sugar. Blood sugar needs to be kept up to the correct level in order to allow both body and mind to function correctly, and the body is very clever at informing us of its requirements. Hence when blood sugar drops below the required level the body sends out signals which are interpreted by the mind as 'I am feeling hungry.' Blood-sugar level is one of the major physical factors in determining the state of hunger. Generally, when the blood-sugar level is high we don't feel hungry – when it is low, we do.

All carbohydrates, sugars and starches are converted into blood sugar. The only difference is that sugars and starches, in the form of refined carbohydrate foods, are more quickly converted into blood sugar. After a meal consisting largely of refined carbohydrate food the blood-sugar level goes up very quickly, which would seem to be a good thing in satisfying the appetite. But then comes the snag.

The body has to have control mechanisms to regulate all its functions. Mechanisms to excrete an appropriate quantity of the water we drink, for instance; otherwise, since we tend to drink so much more than we require, we would eventually burst. Similarly, mechanisms to excrete at least most of the excess salt that we eat, since most of us consume about ten times the amount necessary for our bodily needs.

Blood-sugar level goes up on the digestion of food. But if it were to go up and up and up the blood would become absolutely saturated with sugar which would do us no good at all. Therefore we have a control mechanism to bring down blood-sugar level when it begins to reach unhealthy peaks. This control mechanism involves the substance called insulin, secreted by the pancreas.

When the blood-sugar level shoots up rapidly, the pancreas hurries into action and secretes a large quantity of insulin to keep the situation under control. Insulin in the bloodstream reduces the quantity of blood sugar. All is well for an hour or so. But after about two hours the excess amount of insulin in the blood tends to have an effect which isn't at all helpful to the person seeking to control hunger and food intake. It suppresses the blood-sugar level – not just back to the level before the meal, but even *lower* than the pre-meal level.

This is what is known as rebound hypoglycaemia. On the basis of this scientific fact you can readily understand why many doctors have for years discouraged overweight people from eating carbohydrate-rich foods. However, during all those years of 'cut your carbohydrates' advice, which impressed itself so much on the British public that many people are still overwhelmed with guilt at the sight of a slice of bread or a potato, all high-carbohydrate foods were grouped together as culprits in causing this rebound hunger which led to excessive eating.

More recent research has shown that it is only some carbohydrate foods which cause this problem, not all of them. No prizes for guessing that it is the refined sugary and starchy foods which cause this rebound hunger, and natural fibre-rich foods which do not. The latter are more slowly converted into blood sugar, mainly because of the digestive processes described in the previous chapter. This may well be the reason why the rebound hunger problem does not arise when carbohydrate foods are consumed in their natural fibre-rich form. Whatever the reason, repeated tests have shown that the inclusion of sufficient dietary fibre in meals prevents the excessive output of insulin which so often leads to hunger and snack-eating on diets in which the carbohydrates are processed and refined.

... Yet another reason why dietary fibre helps to control your hunger and your weight.

7

The fibre calorie saving

Once the residue of a meal rich in natural fibre leaves the stomach after its lengthy residence there, it speeds down the intestine at a faster pace. In doing so it saves the dieter from the common curse of constipation, mainly caused by lack of bulk in normal slimming diets. Medical research, which you will read about later in this book, indicates that this faster and more efficient transit may well be helpful in preventing many much more serious illnesses of the lower intestine and bowel, including cancer.

When the faeces are finally expelled, many studies have shown that this waste matter has a higher calorie content than that excreted by people following a normal Western diet containing refined carbo-hydrates.

Happily for most of us, who are inclined to overeat occasionally or frequently, all the calories consumed in food are not used by the body for energy or fat storage. There is a natural wastage of at least five per cent on any diet. But tests so far have clearly shown that dietary fibre increases the wastage and indicated that generally the higher the fibre content the higher the wastage of calories.

In one scientific experiment it was found that a daily increase of 10g of dietary fibre, by the addition of more fruit, vegetables and wholemeal bread to an ordinary Western diet, increased the number of calories excreted in a bowel movement by nearly 90. With still more additional dietary fibre, 32g a day, the stools were found to contain 210 calories on average. However, it must be added that these subjects were consuming quite a large quantity of food and were not attempting to shed weight.

Just why there are more calories in the human excreta following the intake of a high-fibre diet is less than fully understood at the present stage of scientific research. One source of these surplus calories excreted is obviously the non-digestible cell-wall material which forms much of the dietary fibre itself. This is taken into account when calorie figures are given for carbohydrate foods.

Scientific calorie charts, on which all those popular women's magazine calorie charts are based, speak of 'available carbohydrate calories'. This means that the non-digestible calories in the plant cell walls, which will eventually be expelled in the faeces, have already been subtracted in order to give a realistic calorie figure for each carbohydrate food. However, there are other, additional, calories in the faeces expelled after high-fibre eating, in the form of fat and protein. These are not accounted for in the calorie figures. Nor are they fully explained – although less efficient digestion in general is probably a reasonably accurate explanation.

But we have dwelt long enough on this final stage of the fibre slimming story. Suffice it to say that if you are cutting calories in order to shed weight at a speedy pace, every calorie counts. Every calorie that you *don't* make available to your body!

By following a normal mixed 1,000 calorie diet of protein, fat and refined carbohydrate foods you will be making most of those calories available to your body. But you will still shed weight at a good pace. By concentrating on the inclusion of a greater percentage of high-fibre vegetables, fruit and cereal foods in your diet you will be making less of those 1,000 calories available to your body. So you should shed weight at an even faster rate.

The dual aim of most dieters is to become slimmer *and fitter* by following a diet. No one wants to be slim and ill. These days the principal dietary health recommendations of all major nutritional bodies in the Western world are: Eat less fat, less sugar and more dietary fibre. That is precisely what you will do on the F-Plan. Later on in the book we discuss the fitness factor in detail. But now for your guide to losing weight the easy, speedy way – on the F-Plan.

8

How to get the calories right

If you are keeping strictly to 1,000 calories a day and not shedding surplus fat ... then the chances are you are NOT keeping strictly to 1,000 calories a day.

This fact is not intended to hurt anyone's feelings, and still less, dear reader, to cast any aspersions on your honesty and integrity. The truth is that most of us eat (and drink) more calories than we think we are eating (and drinking) in the course of a day. What is more, it is very easy to make mistakes in counting calories. Then there is also that nasty little disorder called 'eating amnesia' which afflicts us all from time to time. Only recently I suffered a modest attack of it myself when recounting what I had eaten, or rather hadn't eaten, that day. 'Mummy,' my son observed after overhearing the conversation, 'if you aren't careful your nose will grow *very*, very long.'

So it is on the basis of us all (EVEN I!) being human and fallible that I have to announce that it is scientifically almost impossible not to shed surplus body fat when calorie intake is strictly limited to 1,000 a day. On the F-Plan it is even less possible – because if you are consuming 1,000 calories a day in the form of fibre-rich meals a percentage of those calories is not digested, as explained in previous chapters. Hence you are providing your body with less than 1,000 calories daily.

My confidence in making the opening statement of this chapter stems not only from scientific fact. Once when I was young, innocent and unaware of eating amnesia, 'weighers-wilt' ('I'll just take a guess at this – looks like two ounces ...!') and other related disorders, I became so alarmed about all the people who couldn't seem to shed weight on 1,000 calories a day that I interviewed many of them, carefully selected a group of twenty of the most baffling and genuine cases, and incarcerated them in a health farm for a week. Then (somewhat sneakily) I had them fed not 1,000 but 1,500 calories daily.

All but two of them shed weight.

The reassuring message from this cautionary tale is that if you are overweight and use the F-Plan calorie tables correctly, as instructed, you simply cannot fail to shed surplus body fat. Health disorders which prevent weight loss are very rare. Almost certainly if you were suffering from such an illness you would have other symptoms to indicate that you were unwell.

The reason why people sometimes think they can't shed weight on a strict calorie ration of 1,000 daily is that they are guessing at the weight – and thus the calorie content – of their portions of food, or forgetting to add in the calories provided by little items like the butter spread on that bread, or the milk in all those cups of tea; or they fail to realize that innocent-looking things like that canned soft drink or glass of orange juice, or the mayonnaise coleslaw served in the office canteen ('Can't contain many calories – it's salad, isn't it!') can add a sizeable number of calories to the daily total.

When people guess at the calorie content of a portion of food they tend to underestimate the calories in meat and cheese, mainly because there was such a deeply entrenched fallacy, persisting for so many years, that 'protein foods' like this could not possibly be fattening. Most people also underestimate the calories provided by fatty foods and fat-containing sauces and dressings. This is simply because the calorie content of these foods is so amazingly high. All fats – butter, margarine, lard, and all the oils including vegetable oils – contain more than 200 calories an ounce. An astronomic figure, when you consider that sugar, for instance, provides, weight for weight, only about half that number of calories, and that potatoes contain only 25 calories an ounce. But again, schooled by the incorrect idea that it is the carbohydrate foods which are the most fattening, many people will very much underestimate the number of calories in the butter-based sauce on their slice of fish, which looks like such an innocent dish.

By the same token, many people *over*estimate the calories provided by potatoes (cooked without fat), cereal foods, and even fat-free sweet foods. Most sweet foods like chocolate, biscuits, cakes and many puddings have a high fat content as well as a high sugar content, so their calorie cost is, indeed, extravagant. However, when sugar is present without much fat or indeed with none, as in a packet of fruit pastilles or some light desserts like crème caramel, the calorie cost is often lower than people imagine.

Of comfort to those of lesser virtue is the fact that pub drinkers, guided only by guesswork, tend to overestimate the calories provided by alcoholic drinks, while innocent orange-juice drinkers, or saintly souls who will 'just stick to a bitter lemon, thanks', often underestimate the number of calories they are consuming. This based on the deeply entrenched conviction that if it looks naughty it must be very fattening, while if it looks innocent or healthy it cannot be. This is not a totally dependable theory when it comes to calorie counting.

I make the distinction of 'pub drinkers' because home drinkers often pour much larger so-called singles and therefore consume *at least* as many calories as they think they are taking in – frequently even more. This applies to spirits rather than wine, for obvious reasons. And, of course, if the bitter-lemon drinker is insisting on one labelled 'low calorie', he or she is consuming hardly any calories at all and is to be congratulated.

From my own observations, made over many years, another great area of calorie error is cold food. We all associate salads with slimming. So if we are eating, for instance, a slice of calorie-crammed quiche surrounded by salad vegetable concoctions oozing with oily or mayonnaisey dressings we are still eating a salad, aren't we, so that can't be very fattening, can it? YES IT CAN. Most people very much underestimate the number of calories in cold salad meals served in restaurants, canteens and cafés.

As you will see from all these examples of overestimating and underestimating, guesswork is dangerous, on the whole, when it comes to calorie counting. I use that qualifying phrase 'on the whole' because there are some foods which allow you to get away with it, some meals in restaurants where you can and indeed have to get away with it, and some people who can get away with it. Let us deal with the people first.

The honest truth, never before revealed, is that there are two types of slimmer. One type can get away with near murder, at least for a while, and still shed some weight. The second type cannot get away with anything, and must keep very precisely to a set number of calories, weighing and measuring food carefully, in order to shed weight. Obviously there must be a third type, hovering somewhere in the middle, but you will be able to work this out for yourself by considering the following characteristics of the two extremes.

The CAN-get-away-with-murder calorie counter: This dieter is heavily overweight (by several stones), large in height as well as bulk.

He or she has been eating a very large quantity of food and has recently embarked on a calorie-counting slimming programme.

Big people who weigh a lot and eat a lot tend to shed weight very easily and speedily when they start cutting down on calorie intake. So even if they are inadvertently or wilfully slipping down a couple of hundred more calories than they intend in the course of a day, they might still find themselves clocking up a decent weight loss on the scales each week.

My message to them: Good luck, and as long as you are satisfied with your weekly weight loss by all means continue to do your own thing. But do be aware that being a little easy-going in working out and rationing your calories can easily allow you to drift down the slippery slope towards being *too* easy-going to achieve weight loss. Such is the frailty of most of our natures that once we take a toe off the straight and narrow we tend to slide off it altogether.

Also, be aware that this happy state of reward for only relative virtue will not continue indefinitely. The body adjusts to lower calorie intake during prolonged periods of dieting, with the result that weight loss tends to slow down. This means that, as we continue to diet, we must reduce calorie intake a little more in order to go on achieving a satisfactory rate of weight loss. This in turn means being even more strict and exact in measuring out the food and counting up the calories. So if your regular weigh-ins start to yield disappointing news, you know what to do.

The CAN'T-get-away-with-anything (darn it!) calorie counter: If you belong to this category you are probably a little person. Things are very unfairly stacked against the short when it comes to slimming. Not only do we display even two or three surplus pounds in the form of an enormous bulge – tall people can often carry a surplus stone without showing it – but we also tend to burn up fewer calories than people of larger height and frame. That means we have to eat less than they do in order to shed weight.

Being only 5′ 2½″ tall myself I too feel very strongly about the unfairness of this, but there is absolutely nothing I can do about it except to warn you that in these circumstances you do need to be very accurate in counting calories in order to achieve a good rate of weight loss. The same applies to anyone, tall or short, who has been dieting for a lengthy period already, and generally to those who are only a few pounds overweight. Weigh, rather than guess, is the general rule to follow in this situation.

Those referred to at the beginning of this chapter, the dieters who think they can't shed weight on 1,000 calories a day, almost invariably belong to the can't-get-away-with-anything group and are not following the essential rules of calorie counting sufficiently strictly. So this is a timely moment to list those rules. Even if you belong to the getting-away-with-murder group, the time will come when you have to follow the rules precisely in order to maintain a speedy weight loss. So here we go:

1. *Be aware that ALL foods, not just some foods, supply calories.* Every single food you see in every supermarket, butcher's, greengrocer's and fishmonger's in the land has calories lurking within. Fibre-rich foods provide calories, too. Because this book explains the many ways in which fibre-rich foods help you to shed weight, I don't want you to imagine that they are calorie-free. In the bad old days of low-carbohydrate diets, many people did, indeed, imagine that those saintly 'protein foods' were calorie-free – I have even known poor souls pouring down vastly fattening cream under the mistaken impression that it was calorie-free because it lacked carbohydrate! Let no similar mistake arise with the F-Plan. The foods which supply you with fibre also supply you with calories. Some of those calories are, in fact, wasted and won't add to your weight. But as we don't yet know how many are wasted, be on the safe side: count the full number given in the F-Plan calorie and fibre charts, and reap the advantage in speed of weight loss.

2. *Weigh your food.* Calories are worked out on a per ounce basis (or in grams, for the modern metric-minded), so how many calories you eat in a portion of food depends on the weight of the portion of food you are eating, WEIGH IT is the key phrase for the calorie-counter. Not weighing it is the key crime. It simply isn't possible to follow a calorie-counting method of slimming without owning some dependably accurate weighing scales – ideally, dietary scales, because with some foods like fats you need to weigh out very small portions.

Most diet advisers sternly insist that you weigh every single thing before putting it in your mouth (cigarettes and fingernails, only, excluded). My own attitude, stemming from a kindly nature, is more permissive. Frankly I think you would look pretty silly weighing out your lettuce when an ounce provides only THREE calories. So what if you go berserk and eat an ounce more lettuce than you think you are eating! Let us be adult about this and accept that, in view of the fact that even the very strictest diets suggest that you eat not much less than 1,000 calories daily, those three calories aren't going to make a jot of difference to your weight loss.

Sometimes the vegetables which are particularly low in calories are not particularly high in fibre. This means they don't do you much good, but neither do they do you any harm. Some vegetables, like cucumber, radishes and lettuce, are mainly water with the occasional vitamin floating around here and there.

Dieters have asked whether they can add these low-calorie vegetables to the meals in the back of the book, and the answer is: Yes. Eat the high-fibre vegetables for their value in health and weight control, but by all means add more variety and colour to your plate, if you wish, with these harmless foods which don't provide enough calories to slow your weight loss.

On the other hand – and this is where many people go wrong – that tiny bit of butter that you sneak onto a crispbread IS going to make a difference because there are such an enormous number of calories in such a very modest quantity of fat. The best tip in using fats like butter, margarine or their lower-calorie alternatives such as Outline or St Ivel Gold is to weigh out half an ounce or an ounce each morning and make that your ready-calorie-counted ration for the day – saves a lot of fiddling around with small quantities. Ditto for the milk you are going to use throughout the day in all those cups of tea and coffee. However, I digress . . .

Earlier in this chapter I explained that with some foods you CAN get away with guesswork about quantity, and weighing is unnecessary. Which foods these are will become clearly evident when you look through the Instant Calorie and Fibre Chart, showing average portions, which starts on page 215. I suggest that where an average portion provides less than 20 calories you let yourself off the chore of weighing while following the F-Plan slimming method. Apart from these, weigh all foods you eat when using the F-Plan calorie and fibre charts.

Listed in Chapter 13 are the meals you can calorie count by guess-work when eating out in restaurants.

3. *Remember that many drinks supply calories, too.* These are every bit as fattening as the calories in solid food, and must be taken into account in reaching your daily total calorie intake. Happily, many drinks are calorie-free or near enough not to matter, and you can drink as much as you like of these (see Chapter 11 and the Drinks Calorie Chart).

I mentioned earlier that it is nearly impossible not to shed surplus weight on a total calorie intake of 1,000 a day when you are following the F-Plan method. I cited that 1,000-calorie total because, to my knowledge, all adults in normal health and circumstances burn up *more* than 1,000 calories daily. Shedding surplus weight depends on providing your body with fewer calories than it needs to keep going. This is the only way in which it can be forced to feed on its own surplus fat. Never believe anything else, whatever silly things you may read or hear elsewhere.

Different bodies have differing calorie requirements to function and fuel their energy output. Size, in both height and weight, is a major factor, and this largely explains why men use more calories than women. The latest scientific investigations into how many calories the average Briton is burning up in this modern labour-saving, sedentary age are yielding somewhat depressing indications.

At one time I would have suggested that everyone would shed surplus fat on a ration of 1,500 calories daily. However, some of my medical and scientific friends now suspect that some women burn up only 1,500 calories daily – so obviously, on this intake, they would maintain weight rather than reduce surplus fat.

However, I am not personally aware of any research revealing that adult British people of either sex or any size can live on 1,000 calories daily without shedding weight, whether they are aiming to do so or not. For this reason 1,000 calories daily is a pretty safe, 'can't fail' figure.

This does not mean, though, that it is the ideal daily calorie quota for every F-Plan dieter. In the next chapter you will find guidance on your own ideal daily calorie ration.

Exercise counts

In answer to a common question from those about to embark on the F-Plan: No, it is not necessary to exercise in order to shed weight. The F-Plan method can make you slim without additional exercises. However, having said that, I am very strongly in favour of increasing physical activity and am among those who suspect that its value in weight control has been much underestimated.

In my experience, the major mistake that dieters make lies in deciding that they *will* exercise once they get slim, rather than starting to increase their physical activity as they start to diet. We had a typical example of this during the F-Plan trials at London University. One attractive but heavily overweight young lady revealed that she spent most of her evenings chatting to friends in a wine bar while dieting. She *did* intend to join a nearby sports club, where she could swim regularly, as soon as she was slim, but meanwhile shyly admitted to feeling too embarrassed to be seen in a swimsuit.

The situation arising from this all-too-common attitude was as follows: in the evening she was placing herself in a situation of maximum temptation as far as diet-breaking was concerned – with time on her hands and food and drink all too readily available. There is nothing quite as bad as watching other people eat and drink what you are trying to avoid. Had she embarked on an evening swim instead, she would have achieved all these advantages in helping her to keep to her diet:

1. She would have been kept busy and occupied, and well away from the sight, smell and temptation of food.

2. She would have experienced the undoubted lift in spirits that results from physical exercise. Depressed moods are the most difficult moods for dieting, and such is the mood-lifting effect of exercise that it is even being used medically as part of the treatment for depression.

3. She would have burned up extra calories, thus helping to speed her weight loss still more.

4. She would have experienced that glow of virtue which is so conducive to easy dieting. When we feel pleased with our achievements we tend to feel inspired to achieve even more in the way of health and figure improvement.

I am very well aware of the sensitivity of anyone who is overweight. It can often arise even when people are a mere few pounds overweight. But if you are contemplating increasing physical activity for still further benefit to your health and figure, try to realize that those vast crowds of people who will scream with laughter at the sight of you in a swimsuit, or on seeing you jogging, skipping, enrolling at aerobics classes or even taking a brisk daily walk, exist only in your mind. The best time to start exercising is at the start rather than at the end of a dieting campaign.

9

Calories: how low can you go?

Hunger is a problem that simply should not arise on the F-Plan, even though you are restricting the actual number of calories consumed each day. This does not mean that you cannot possibly be tempted by the sight of a chocolate bar or the scent of a fish and chip shop, but you will more easily be able to resist. Because the calories consumed are in the form of particularly bulky, filling and satisfying food your appetite will not be sharpened nor your willpower lowered by actual physical hunger.

We live in a world where food temptations flaunt themselves all around us. They pop up in the commercials on the TV screen, on the usherette's tray at the cinema, in every other shop window. In the Western world, unless you are sitting in a canoe in the middle of the Atlantic it is almost impossible to be far from the sight of food. Even in that situation you would probably be rescued by a passing cruise ship, on board which they would stuff you endlessly with food to compensate for the boredom of the interminable view of the sea. Food, in our society, is used for many reasons other than simply to satisfy hunger. It is used for comfort, pleasure, socializing, celebrating, time-filling, seduction – to name just a few of the alternatives.

Obviously, the person who is not actually hungry is considerably less vulnerable to the temptations of our food-filled Western world. Psychiatrists studying shopping behaviour have found – not surprisingly – that the hungry woman is much more inclined to succumb to impulse food buys. She generally fills her supermarket trolley more fully when she shops just before a meal than if she shops shortly after one, when her hunger is fully satisfied. Supermarket chiefs, always seeking new ways to cram more food down us, would be wise to offer a special shop-before-lunch discount!

When you are eating a fibre-rich diet there are restraining limits on how many calories you can actually manage to consume in a day – even if you aren't trying to shed weight. This was illustrated most illuminatingly by a recent study in which a group of people were asked to eat more than a pound of potatoes each day (baked in their skins, not fried) in addition to whatever other food they could manage to eat. By adding these potatoes, a bulky food of reasonably high-fibre content, they actually lost some weight over a three-month period! The potatoes were so filling that there wasn't a great deal of room left for all the other foods they usually ate.

This was impressive. But it certainly wouldn't be fair to claim that all you need to do in order to shed surplus weight is to add sufficient fibre-rich foods to your diet – or switch from refined carbohydrate foods to natural fibre-rich foods like wholemeal bread.

In the future, when you have become slim, the change from refined carbohydrate foods to their high-fibre alternatives should be sufficient to keep you that way. Certainly it will do so if you also put some restraints on your intake of fats. This is clearly indicated by the natural slenderness of those among the Third World societies who live on plentiful supplies of foods high in fibre content. So the F-Plan does have a great stay-slim bonus. Food preferences are very much dictated by habit, and those who get into the habit of choosing the fibre-rich foods gradually come to prefer them.

However, most people aiming to shed surplus weight are also aiming to do so reasonably swiftly. To be frank, the basic aim of most dieters is to shed two tons of weight by yesterday! This attitude is understandable, and slimming experts who drearily continue to tell us to 'be satisfied just to lose weight slowly: half a pound a week is enough' have little or no understanding of human psychology.

The F-Plan requires less actual effort than any other slimming diet you have followed before. But all slimming diets – the F-Plan included – require some degree of conscious effort and self-control. In order to sustain effort, in this and all other areas of life, we need the feedback of reward – ideally, short-term reward rather than some far distant pot of gold, way off at the end of the rainbow. The essential reward for the dieter is that weekly weight loss. There are few joys in life to compare with that of stepping on the scales and discovering that you weigh measurably less this week than you did last.

A miserable half pound is barely recordable. Any seasoned dieter knows full well that she can 'cheat' that weight off the normal set of bathroom scales by shifting her stance a little or rushing off to empty the bladder, remove the dentures and so on. Yes, don't think we weren't watching you . . . A measurable weight loss needs to be at least in the region of 2lb a week in order to provide that reward so essential to sustained effort. You can't 'cheat' off 2lb! In slimming, success tends to breed success and vice versa. Every slimming club leader knows that it is the member who registers a good weight loss at her weekly weigh-in who is most likely to keep up her dieting and return to the club next week, while the member who records a disappointingly low weight loss is the most likely to drop out. In dieting, failure does not make us try harder. Usually, it makes us give up.

On the F-Plan we are aiming for an average weekly weight loss in the region of 3lb in order to keep spirits up as weight goes down. The loss could well be considerably higher, particularly if you are male or heavily overweight; but over-high expectations can be just as demoralizing as very slow weight loss, so we are taking a restrained attitude.

On the F-Plan the calories will be consumed in food which is more filling, and your body will waste more of them than on other slimming diets. However, we recommend that you keep to the usual recommended calorie intakes for weight loss, and reap the additional advantages in ease and speed, rather than try to eat even fewer calories than usually recommended in a diet. Remember, most dieters fail to stay the course. The F-Plan's extra filling power can most help you by getting you right to slim-weight target. The 'easy' diet is the one that succeeds, because it is the one you continue to follow until you are slim.

Frankly, the only people I can think of who need to go as low as 850 calories a day in order to achieve a pacey weight loss on the F-Plan are small, rather sedentary women, only a few pounds overweight, and those struggling off the last few pounds of excess weight after a prolonged dieting campaign. In these circumstances, increasing energy expenditure helps, too – by which I mean generally moving around as much as possible, doing a lot of brisk walking and speeding this up to running pace if you are young.

To shed surplus weight with the F-Plan, allow yourself a maximum of 1,500 calories a day and a minimum of 1,000 calories (or less only if medically supervised) a day. You may choose to set your daily calorie intake anywhere between those two limits. These recommendations will guide you to your own ideal daily calorie limits for successful weight loss.

Allow yourself 1,500 calories daily

* If you are male, of at least medium height, and more than half a stone overweight. Men have a greater daily calorie requirement than women, so they can shed weight on more generous slimming diets and generally record considerably larger weekly weight losses. This is unfair, but something that even Women's Liberation cannot change. Few men could fail to shed weight at a satisfactory rate on a daily allowance of 1,500 calories.

* If you are female, more than two stones overweight, and just embarking on a weight-loss programme – as opposed to switching from another slimming diet on which you have already lost some of your surplus weight. The more heavily overweight people are, the more swiftly they can shed surplus fat on a slimming diet. This rate of loss tends to slow down as weight goes down and the metabolism adjusts, to some degree, to dieting. So if you are starting out with a good deal of weight to shed, it is wise to allow scope for reducing calorie intake in the later stages of dieting. Start on 1,500 calories daily, and work your way gradually down to 1,000 daily in order to maintain a good, encouraging rate of loss.

Set your daily calorie intake between 1,000 and 1,500 (if you wish) by taking into account the following:

These factors tend to increase speed of weekly weight loss on a diet
* Being male.
* Being heavily overweight.
* Being at the start of a slimming programme, rather than at a midway stage.
* Being in the habit of eating a generous quantity of food – the more you have been eating the greater the initial weight loss impact when you switch to a slimming diet.
* Being involved in a job which necessitates a good deal of physical

activity (housework, unfortunately, does not rate high in this way, in these days of mod. cons.), or taking part in a good deal of sport or walking (that ten-minute daily dozen doesn't really rate here, either).

Allow yourself 1,000 calories daily

* If you are a small man, with only a few pounds of surplus weight, and are in a big hurry to lose it.
* If you are female and less than one stone overweight.
* If you are female and more than a stone overweight, but have already been dieting and have lost a stone or more on any other slimming method.

Reduce calorie intake to 850 if you must, but ONLY in these circumstances:

* If you are just thinking in terms of an occasional day, maybe a couple of days a week. Our desire for food tends to vary from day to day. On some days it is easy to eat very little, on others it is difficult to keep to even the most generous diet. It seems sensible to take advantage of the good days in order to make allowance for any excess eating on the difficult days, and dieting calorie intake can be averaged out on a weekly basis. If you eat more on some days and less on others, you will shed weight just as successfully as if you stuck to the same number of calories each day.

* If you are only planning to follow the F-Plan for a week or two to polish off a modest weight problem of just a few pounds. If you have been following a normal varied British pattern of eating you have probably been consuming less dietary fibre than you need for health protection, but it is unlikely that you are deficient in minerals and vitamins. In those circumstances, vitamin and mineral deficiencies do not crop up in a couple of weeks. However, on a calorie intake of below 1,000 a day it is a reasonable idea to take a multi-vitamin pill with iron – just to keep your mother, and me, happy.

These factors tend to slow speed of weight loss on a diet

*   Being female.
*   Being only a few pounds overweight.
*   Being at the tail-end of a slimming campaign. Those last few pounds can prove the most stubborn, but the F-Plan will help.
*   Having a naturally restrained appetite, which probably means that you are only a few pounds overweight and have gained this weight over a lengthy period. We all think we eat less than we do!
*   Being a sedentary type of person. This doesn't just mean doing a sedentary job but refers rather to the type of person (who could well be a housewife, doing a basically non-sedentary type of job) who calls the children to bring something from the next room rather than getting up herself, or who goes to great lengths to avoid journeys up and down stairs, or who will drive round for five minutes to find a parking spot near the exit of the car park rather than walk for two minutes . . . The sum total of all those little movements makes a big difference to daily calorie expenditure and varies a good deal among individuals. The people who move a good deal are often described as being 'full of nervous energy'. It is not the so-called 'nervous' aspect that burns up the calories, but the frequent physical movement. These always-on-the-move people are usually slim.

10

Fibre: how high can you go?

Although statistics on dietary fibre intake were not recorded until 1919, the Royal College of Physicians thinks it probable that it has halved in Britain since the middle of the last century.

Today, the average intake of 20g a day puts us among the lowest fibre-consumers in the world. Indeed, it is quite difficult to find nations who eat less dietary fibre than the British, apart from the Swedes (14g daily) and Masai warriors, who are thought to eat practically none! U.S. citizens score a little higher than we do, with an average intake of 27g daily. But this is still modest compared with the quantity thought to have been consumed by our ancestors and the quantity being consumed, today, by societies in the underdeveloped world.

Surveys of these societies sometimes reveal remarkably high intake figures – 130g a day among the Kikuyu of Kenya and a staggering 150g daily among the Buganda of Uganda, for instance. Generally, however, people of the poorer African and Asian countries consume two to three times our quantity of fibre. Their intake of 40g to 60g daily is thought, by many medical experts and eminent medical authorities, to be highly significant in relation to the fact that major killers of the Western world, like cancer of the bowel and heart disease, are virtually unknown in these high fibre consuming societies. And so is obesity!

Just because you are British you can't even assume you are eating your 20g a day. This is an average figure. Individual variations are great. Surveys show that some Britons are consuming as little as 6g daily. What is worse, if you are concerned about your excess weight you are likely to be among the lower consumers of dietary fibre. Studies have indicated that the weight conscious, brainwashed by years of 'cut out those carbohydrates' advice, tend to avoid the bread and potatoes which supply a good deal of the fibre in most people's diets.

Dieting and nutritional fallacies die hard. As you embark on the F-Plan you might have to work quite energetically to convince yourself that the supposed virtues of the old low-carbohydrate method of dieting have been disproved by recent research. Medical experts no longer approve of this method of dieting – largely because of the limits it places on the intake of cereals, fruit and root vegetables. Bread (if it is wholemeal!) and potatoes are no longer considered the baddies in health and obesity. Fats and sugars have revealed themselves as the real villains.

And, when you think about it, did *you* succeed in getting permanently slim by struggling to cut out carbohydrates for all those years?

When you follow the F-Plan menus you can hardly fail to increase daily dietary fibre intake considerably – even if you don't bother to count the grams.

The average Briton's full daily intake of 20g is provided by the two pieces of fruit, and muesli-type mix called Fibre-Filler, which you are required to eat each day as part of this slimming plan. ALL the meals, from which you can choose freely, have been specially devised to contain a good percentage of those foods which supply a significant quantity of dietary fibre.

You should find it easy to consume 35g of fibre daily, and we suggest this as the lower limit in order to achieve the slimming benefits described in the previous chapters. Those keeping to a strict 1,000 calories a day allowance will usually find this to be a realistic target. Obviously, if you are eating more fibre-rich food you are likely to eat more grams of fibre. Those allowing themselves 1,500 calories daily might reach a fibre intake of 50g daily. We advise this as the higher limit.

If, after reading the advice in Chapter 9, you decide to keep to a very strict calorie intake of just 850 to 1,000 calories daily, you will find it very difficult to achieve the upper levels of the fibre recommendation and might even find it difficult to consume 35 grams of fibre daily. Don't worry. In these circumstances 30 grams daily will suffice. You are, you see, still consuming a very high *percentage* of dietary fibre. The average Briton who is not attempting to shed weight is consuming between 2,000 and 3,000 calories daily and only around 15 to 20 grams of fibre. So you will be taking in about twice as much dietary fibre in less than half as much food. You are on a high-fibre diet even on 30 grams a day. So the recommendations are a helpful guideline, not a biblical edict. No need to get too fussed about the odd gram.

All the meals on the F-Plan menu are fibre-counted for you. Don't worry about small day-to-day variations in intake, or aim for precise rounded figures – simply choose your menus to provide between 35g and 50g of dietary fibre each day.

11

What (and how much) to drink

On the F-Plan you are asked to drink a generous amount of calorie-free liquid, but only a very modest quantity of calorie-supplying liquid.

One liquid is obligatory. You must have half a pint of skimmed milk each day. This is to help ensure nutritional balance in your diet and, in particular, to supply calcium, because dietary fibre can hinder the absorption of calcium to some degree. There is no evidence of health problems arising from this particular factor, but on this healthy diet we want to take extra care to ensure all essential nutrients. You will also need to use at least part of this milk with your cereal breakfasts.

Doctors who prescribe high-fibre diets for health problems sometimes advocate a generous daily intake of fluid. One of the aims and functions of a high-fibre diet is to sustain a large bulk of semi-fluid matter in the stomach, and to produce more soft and bulky faeces. The fibre itself will ensure this but the extra fluid may help it a little – certainly the fluid has to come from somewhere, and it will do no harm if it is calorie-free. Calorie-free fluids do not add to body fat, hinder weight loss or cause fluid retention in those of normal health. The idea that they do so is one of the most persistent slimming myths of all.

Neither – to put another old fallacy to rest – is drinking with meals 'fattening', if the drinks are calorie-free. Drinking with meals the correct way can actually be 'slimming', in that it can helpfully add to the time it takes to consume high-fibre meals. The right way is to put down knife and fork in order to take a sip of water (or other calorie-free liquid) after a mouthful of food has been chewed and swallowed. The wrong, or 'fattening' way, to drink with meals is to use the drink to swill food down the throat before it has been swallowed, because then it will speed rather than slow the ingestion of food.

The reason why you are asked to be restrained in drinking calorific drinks is that these, even more than refined carbohydrate foods, have the opposite effect from fibre-rich foods in nearly all those steps in the consumption process which influence your degree of hunger. While fibre-rich foods are chewed slowly, calorific drinks require no chewing at all and go down the throat in a split second. While fibre-rich foods fill the stomach for lengthy periods, calories supplied in fluid alone pass through more quickly than any digested from solid foods.

Observers of eating behaviour have noted that people can take in very large numbers of calories in the form of liquids without noticeably diminishing their appetite for food at all.

Please read the following very important instructions about drinking while you are following the F-Plan.

Daily milk allowance

Your daily half pint of milk must be skimmed milk. This is essential. Half a pint of skimmed milk provides just 100 calories, while other kinds of milk can provide twice this number. Don't buy silver-top and skim off the cream yourself, because this doesn't provide an equivalent calorie saving. These days most dairies will deliver skimmed milk, so ask the milkman if he can supply it. Many supermarkets sell cartons of skimmed milk, sometimes sensibly labelled 'for slimmers'. You can also buy skimmed milk in powdered form; Marvel is one such product. So skimmed milk is now easily available, since people have become more aware of the dangerously fattening potential of full-cream milk.

Calorie-free drinks

All the following drinks are calorie-free, or negligible in calories, so they can be consumed freely on the F-Plan: water; tea and black coffee (without sugar, of course, though you can add milk from your daily half-pint allowance); all bottled drinks like bitter lemon, Diet Pepsi and Tab which are specially labelled 'low calorie'. These days most major manufacturers of non-alcoholic beverages produce special drinks of negligible calorie content for the weight-conscious. These include Canada Dry mixers, Energen one-calorie Drinks, Hunt's low-calorie mixers, Schweppes Slimline range, and Chekwate, Concorde, Safeway, Sunfresh, Tesco and Waitrose low-calorie drinks. But do check for that low-calorie label.

Of course the fashionable mineral waters – Perrier, Evian, Vichy, Malvern, and so on – are calorie-free, and are becoming increasingly popular in smart restaurants. So you can be chic as you get slim!

Bovril and Oxo do supply a few calories, but too few to be worth counting, and can provide a nice, hot, comforting drink on a dieting evening.

Real fruit juices

Fruit juices, other than lemon juice, are *not* allowed on the F-Plan. This is one of the ways in which this new method differs from diets of the past. The reason is that fruit juices are simply fruit stripped of its natural fibre content. When you drink orange juice you are getting all the calories which are present in the orange in the form of sugar, but with none of the fibre filling power. When you buy a small can of frozen concentrated orange juice you are getting the fibre-free contents of a large quantity of oranges, at a cost of more than 200 calories per can. Many people could easily consume a full can, diluted, during a thirsty summer day, and it would have little if any effect in reducing an appetite for solid food. To consume the same quantity of calories in the form of whole oranges you would have to eat about five of them. Obviously this would have some realistic effect in satisfying the appetite.

Manufacturers are doing the weight-prone no favour in removing fibre from fruits to make them into juices. Scientific tests recorded a great reduction in satiety level when subjects were fed apple juice (apples with their fibre removed) compared with the same quantity of apples eaten whole. The apple juice speeded the fibre-stripped apple through the mouth and stomach and also raised the blood-sugar level in a way which led to the rebound hunger factor described in a previous chapter. The apples produced all the weight-control benefits of low ingestion, high bulk and a lengthy period in the stomach – and they did not lead to rebound hunger.

By getting used to eating oranges rather than drinking orange juice, eating apples rather than drinking apple juice, and so on, you are establishing a good habit which will help to control your weight in the future.

Fruit-juice production is one of the 'refining' processes which can unfortunately help to increase our intake of calories on a modern Western diet. Lemon juice, however, unlike other fruit juices, is virtually calorie-free, as it lacks the sugar present in the juice of other fruit. Obviously you would need to sweeten this unless you have very eccentric taste buds – but saccharin sweeteners can do the job without calorie cost – making it an acceptable drink.

Alcohol

As far as health, fitness and fast weight loss are concerned, it is obviously better to avoid alcohol while following the F-Plan or any other slimming diet.

However, those are all physical factors. There are psychological factors to be taken into account, too. If you feel deprived and miserable by not being allowed an early evening drink, or a glass of wine with your evening meal, it is usually better to allow yourself a little alcohol while dieting. Otherwise it is unlikely that you are going to keep to the diet for very long. However, here is the vital F-Plan rule:

If you are allowing yourself a daily ration of alcohol, allow these calories in addition to a minimum calories' worth of food and milk from the F-Plan menus. First, allow 100 calories from the half pint of skimmed milk, and another 100 calories for your daily apple and orange. Then make up a minimum of 650 calories (more, if you are allowing yourself between 1,000 and 1,500 a day) from Fibre-Filler (see page 65) and the meals on the F-Plan menus. After that you can add the appropriate number of calories from alcohol.

Nearly everyone, female as well as male, can shed surplus fat at a good pace on 1,250 calories a day, and the vast majority of people will achieve a satisfactory weight loss on 1,500 calories a day. So nearly everyone can afford to drink a little alcohol while they are dieting, if they wish.

Alcohol does not provide any useful nutrients or fibre; hence the reason for consuming all your daily calories from food and milk, to ensure good nutrition, before adding any 'empty' alcoholic calories.

If preferred, calories can be averaged out on a weekly rather than a daily basis. For instance, as long as you average 8,750 calories a week you will shed weight just as quickly by having as many as 1,870 a day on Saturdays and Sundays, and only 1,000 each weekday, as you would by counting precisely 1,250 calories a day for all seven days of the week. This fact can be used to advantage by those who drink alcohol occasionally – perhaps only once or twice a week on social occasions, and not every day. Obviously, in terms of calories you can afford to drink a greater quantity of alcohol if it is an occasional rather than a daily indulgence.

You will find that the Drinks Calorie Guide (page 276) provides a very realistic way of measuring the calories consumed in the form of alcoholic drinks.

12

Fibre-Filler, the F-Plan's inbuilt slimming aid

While following the F-Plan you will be able to choose from a wide variety of meals to suit your own taste, in selecting daily menus. Nevertheless to make it really easy to reach your daily dietary fibre target of 30g plus, it is an excellent idea to have one regular, constant daily meal – breakfast is ideal because we tend not to vary our breakfasts – to supply about half the requirement. Add a couple of pieces of fruit each day as part of your menu, and after that it isn't at all difficult to include enough dietary fibre in your other two meals to succeed in your aims.

One of the great successes of the F-Plan method has been such a meal, a kind of home-made muesli, called Fibre-Filler. We think you will be surprised at the remarkable effect this relatively modest-looking quantity of food will have in satisfying your appetite for really long periods.

Your daily portion of Fibre-Filler provides 15g of dietary fibre, which is more than many Britons normally consume in a day. Most of this fibre is from cereal sources which are particularly recommended for their health value by some leading medical researchers. But fibre from fruit and nut sources is included too, which adds health and slimming value.

To make your daily quantity of Fibre-Filler, mix together the following ingredients:

For one day

½oz Bran Flakes
½oz bran
½oz All Bran or Bran Buds
¼oz almonds, chopped
¼oz dried prune (just one large fruit), stoned and chopped
¼oz dried apricots, chopped
½oz sultanas

Obviously you will find it easier to multiply the ingredients and make several daily servings at one time. But if you do, mix the ingredients well (the bran tends to filter down to the bottom, in its dry state), divide into daily quantities and store in separate plastic storage bags.

For eight days:

4oz Bran Flakes
4oz bran
4oz All Bran or Bran Buds
2oz almonds, chopped
2oz dried prunes, stoned and chopped
2oz dried apricots, chopped
4oz sultanas

Your daily quantity of Fibre-Filler tastes surprisingly good once you have mixed it with milk. If you like muesli-type cereals, you will find the taste pleasing. What is more, although the quantity for the day looks relatively modest in dry state, once it is mixed with milk you will find that it provides two good and satisfying servings.

We recommend that one serving (half the daily quantity) should be used to provide breakfast and a highly satisfying start to the day. This should keep you comfortably free of hunger right through to lunch.

The remaining half of the Fibre-Filler plays an equally helpful role in aiding willpower. Save this to be eaten at any time during the day (in addition to your other meals) when you begin to feel hungry and vulnerable to eating temptations. Many people will decide to save it until suppertime. Evenings represent maximum temptation for most slimmers, although around four o'clock in the afternoon, when the children come home from school, can be the worst time for many mothers who may be waiting until mid evening to dine with their husbands. In these circumstances, this might be the best time to eat the remaining portion.

Yet another way in which you might choose to use the second half of your daily Fibre-Filler is to divide it into two portions and eat one of these half an hour before each of the two main meals of the day. This way it will act rather like an appetite suppressant pill – or, rather, in the way pills should act if they contained sufficient cellulose. Fibre-Filler does contain a generous quantity of cellulose, so you will be feeling considerably less hungry when you start each meal; you will be able to eat more slowly and be very satisfied with a diet-restricted quantity of food.

The daily Fibre-Filler, made in the quantities given here, provides a total of 200 calories. These should be subtracted from your total allowance of 850 to 1,500 calories for the day.

Milk used with Fibre-Filler should be taken from the daily half pint of skimmed milk. You will find that only a small quantity of milk is necessary and that a quarter of a pint is quite sufficient to accompany the full daily Fibre-Filler allowance – an eighth of a pint with each portion. This will leave you a quarter of a pint of milk for tea and coffee through the day.

It is unlikely you will find Fibre-Filler unpalatable. It is a most important and valuable part of the F-Plan programme, so do include it. However, for occasional days when you might find yourself caught out with no time or ingredients (try to plan ahead to avoid this: you can easily carry Fibre-Filler with you in a plastic bag in your handbag!) we have listed a few alternative very high fibre breakfasts in The F-Plan Meals.

Ideally, breakfast on half your daily portion of Fibre-Filler or have it mid morning if you dislike eating early in the day. Only when this is not possible should you have one of the alternative high-fibre breakfasts.

13

Eating out on the F-Plan

The F-Plan provides you with many easy-to-carry meals, like sandwiches, and, hopefully, you will take your lunch to work with you while dieting.

However, business lunches may crop up from time to time – and also evening invitations which involve dining at restaurants. It is somewhat unrealistic to expect to retire completely from social life. It is quite insane to imagine that you are going to sit in a restaurant adding up calories and grams of fibre. This is also quite impossible – nearly all restaurant meals are very low in fibre content and nearly every dish varies in calorie content from restaurant to restaurant.

So what are we to do?

The answer is simply to use the common-sense approach and avoid making the mistakes which cost the average slimmer so many unsuspected calories while eating out.

Forget about fibre while dining out. With your stomach nicely fibre-full from other meals you should not, at least, arrive at the restaurant table like a ravenous wolf. So this should help you in keeping the calorie intake low. To do so follow two simple guidelines.

1. Keep to the low-fat dishes.
2. Keep to the very simple dishes.

The first guideline is very important, not only for reducing your weight now but for controlling it in the future. The weight-conscious so often choose the most fattening dishes on the menu, in the mistaken idea that they were being virtuous. No, no ... they would not *dream* of having potatoes or a dessert. But they will select dishes absolutely swimming in butter or choose cheese instead of dessert. Fats are by far the most fattening foods of all. Even those tiny little protein-packed escargots or that leafy garden-of-Eden innocent asparagus or artichoke can be calorie-packed because of the luscious lure of all that horrifically high-calorie butter.

The old, and now much condemned, low-carbohydrate method of dieting had much to answer for in making social eaters fat. The idea that 'if it isn't sugary or starchy it can't be fattening' has accounted for the eating of many excess calories in restaurants.

Now, thanks to the publicity of the past year or two, people are beginning to realize that fats are dieters' enemy number one. Fats are more than twice as fattening as any other food. F-Plan dieters know that high-fibre carbohydrate foods are dieters' friend number one – they are the pioneers of a completely new and more effective attitude to food and weight control. But those old ideas do take a long time to die.

The reason for guideline number two, 'keep to the very simple dishes', is that fats can lurk in disguise in all kinds of sauce-covered dishes or recipe dishes. Did you know that taramasalata is crammed with fat? Or that avocado is the only fat-containing fruit – and that when you order it with an oily dressing, or with prawns in mayonnaise dressing, you are ordering one of the most fattening first courses of all? With that, or taramasalata, or pâté (also usually high in fat content), you could well be packing down more than 400 calories before you even start your main course.

That nasty shock should emphasize the importance of low-fat simplicity in restaurant meals while dieting.

All sauces, mayonnaise and salad dressings, creamed soups and cheese-containing concoctions should be considered highly suspect sources of excess calories. And Heaven knows the calorie mysteries of the East! Do you know how many calories are in Mr Singh's curry or Mr Wong's sweet-and-sour? Quite inscrutable, of course. Better give exotic Eastern eating a miss, if you are aiming at shedding weight fast.

Keep to the safest, simplest dishes when eating in restaurants while you follow the F-Plan slimming diet. Here is the regrettably modest list of best bets in each course.

Starters	Maximum calorie total per serving

These are the only really dependably low-calorie choices:

Consommé – any flavour (lovely and clear, so you can actually *see* that they have not sneaked in extra calories)	60

Oysters (for rich readers), each	5
Half a grapefruit (for poor readers)	20
A slice of melon, any kind	40
Any fresh fruit cocktail	60
Smoked salmon (if you can eat it 'neat' without *buttered* bread)	80
Parma ham with melon (a little more calorie-costly – but they are usually providentially mean with the ham), don't eat the ham fat	150

Main courses	Maximum calorie total per serving

Grilled Dover sole (not buttery), be assertive about any plain grilled white fish, tell the waiter that you do not want it served swimming with butter. Send it back if it is	350
Grilled liver (waiter's instructions as above)	250
Lobster, without one of those rich sauces (again, we give sensitive consideration to the problems of rich readers)	200
Plain grilled steak (6oz) with salad	300
Any seafood – crab, prawns, etc. – with salad (but be risqué! Insist that the salad is served totally undressed. If you add dressing, be very, very mean with it)	100
Omelettes (you cannot go too far wrong with an omelette, unless it is made with cheese, so no cheese, please)	350

Any vegetables can be ordered with these dishes, as long as you are sure they are not cooked or served with fat. A baked potato is very permissible, of course. But, without your low-calorie dressing to hand (you could smuggle it in a hip flask, perhaps), order a baked potato in restaurants only if you can resist that terribly high-calorie sour cream or butter. Be honest with yourself about this – rather than optimistic.

Desserts	Maximum calorie total per serving

The choice here is very simple. Ideally choose any fresh fruit – raspberries (fibre-high as well as calorie-low), strawberries, fresh figs, fresh fruit salad, but all without the cream, please. For those yearning for something just a little more sinful, the following are also dependably calorie-low:

Any fresh fruit sorbets	100
Crème caramel (when the waiter asks 'with cream, madame?' the answer is 'No')	200
Ice cream (but only if it is a simple, honest old-fashioned ice – not one of those staggeringly exotic multi-storey jobs, rising with layer upon layer of heaven-knows-what and terminating with a big blob of shaving cream)	150

Do not have cheese instead of a dessert. Most cheeses are crammed with fat and horribly high in calories.

14

The startling truth about US and THEM

The British are not, on the whole, all that keen on health. Of course, we worry about good health if we don't enjoy it. But if we do appear to be reasonably well . . . well then, what is there to concern ourselves about? The national worry quota is already more than filled to overflowing by income tax, Ken Livingstone and all those disturbing goings-on in *Coronation Street*.

Certainly, people-maintenance is not the national preoccupation in Britain that it is in America. There, as many an unwary traveller has discovered to his cost, the major hazard on the sidewalks is not muggers and rapists, but the imminent danger of being trampled to death by the endless stream of passing joggers. In many ways, they have replaced the buffalo.

Tea-time (sorry, coffee-time) chat in America is full of phrases like 'chemical additives', which they are generally against. And while we have been making a resolution every New Year's Eve for the past forty years to attend exercise classes – and most certainly *will* get around to it some time during the next thirty – they actually *do*. Really! Many American women honestly do attend exercise classes, not just once a week but sometimes several times. There are actually women like American *Cosmopolitan*'s editor, Helen Gurley Brown, who spend more than an hour of every busy day doing exercises. The thought is quite exhausting enough to make us lie down and take a nap.

To be fair, there are two groups of Britons who are very concerned about health maintenance. The first, known as cranks, tend to swallow some extraordinary theories. The second, known as hypochondriacs, tend to swallow a large number of useless potions purchased from over the chemist's counter. But these are just two little subcultures, and in no way representative of Britain as a whole.

The Americans are very concerned about health. We are generally unconcerned about health. But, on both sides of the Atlantic, we can congratulate ourselves and count on our good fortune in having all the benefits of modern medicine to protect us – unlike the peoples of the undeveloped world.

Many of us are old enough to remember the days when to contract tuberculosis — which many British people did — was to be given a virtual death sentence. This was still the situation as recently as the 1940s. Now, TB is practically non-existent in the Western world, and something we tend to forget all about, except on the odd cultural occasion when we hear Mimi coughing herself so touchingly and melodically to death in *La Bohème*, or read the life of a Lakeland poet, or dwell on the saga of the Lady of the Camellias. All the best people, it seemed, used to die of 'consumption' — as it was then called. And large numbers of ordinary people as well used to die of TB. Until recently it was one of the greatest of all killer diseases.

If you are in your forties you can also flash your mind back to those dramatic posters: 'Diphtheria is deadly — protect your child by immunization', and probably recall some child at your school who contracted polio and was crippled for life.

One of the most marvellous happenings of the past few decades is the way in which infective diseases have been brought under control and even virtually abolished by modern drugs and vaccines, better hygiene, safe water supplies, modern sewage systems.

IN THE WESTERN WORLD . . . that is. People in undeveloped African and Asian countries do not have all our modern advantages and some infective diseases, which have become part of history here, remain rampant there. As the charity organizations keep reminding us, millions of people continue to die in Africa and Asia from diseases which are both preventable and curable. No wonder that poor people living in the traditional way in India and many African countries have a considerably shorter life expectancy than we — with our better living conditions and easily available medicine.

Or do they?

Prepare yourself for a major shock to your assumptions. It is true that a comparison of the generally accepted life-expectancy figures between the West and the Third World countries, or a comparison between ourselves and our grandparents' generation, would show that modern Western man has a great advantage in *average* expectation of life. But these figures are highly deceptive. Largely the difference is accounted for by a dramatic decrease in child mortality in the modern Western world, due to vast improvements in hygiene, protection against infective disease and plentiful food. In many Third World countries as many as three out of five children die before the age of five. Wander around any English country churchyard and you will see that here, too, child mortality was very common in the past, even at the start of the century. When life-expectancy figures are calculated, everyone who has been born and died is taken into account in arriving at the average life-expectancy figures. Obviously, the short lives of all those babies and children will have a great effect in bringing down the average figure – as even the least mathematical of us will be able to understand.

Those who are born in the Third World have a considerably smaller chance of surviving childhood than those born here – and the same was true of those born in the West a hundred years ago. There is an enormous difference in the child-mortality figures.

But what of the expectation of life of someone who has reached the age of forty?

It may surprise you to discover that the continued life expectancy of a forty-year-old man in Britain today has scarcely increased at all on that of a forty-year-old man living in Britain a century ago. Having conquered the killer epidemics of infectious diseases it seems strange that we do not have a greater life expectancy in this sense too.

Considering the rifeness of disease, the poverty and the malnutrition prevalent there, and all the medical aid available here, it is even more surprising to discover that the continued life expectancy of a forty-year-old British or US citizen is not considerably greater than that of an Indian who has survived childhood and reached the age of forty. This is true of the inhabitants of most of the undeveloped Third World countries.

Both in America, where they are much more concerned with health, and in Britain, where we tend to take health for granted until it becomes a problem, the general pattern is that we are rattling through merrily until our forties and fifties, and then . . .

The middle-aged are being afflicted by a great plague of modern Western illnesses, many of them fatal. These illnesses are not caught from germs and viruses. They seem to creep up on us gradually – for reasons that medical science is only now beginning to understand. They are known, collectively, as degenerative diseases.

Among the major degenerative diseases is coronary heart disease, the commonest cause of death in Western countries, killing about one man in four. The second great destroyer is cancer – cancer of the lung and cancer of the bowel being the most common fatal forms of cancer in Britain.

As well as the two 'big Cs', coronaries and cancer, there is a whole group of other degenerative diseases like diabetes, diverticulosis and other disorders of the bowel – and less serious but still troublesome problems like varicose veins, haemorrhoids and constipation.

The big factor that all these illnesses and health problems have in common is that they are virtually non-existent among Third World communities, living on what-grows-naturally in age-old traditional ways. However, when groups from such communities move to and settle in countries living and eating in Western style, and adopt Western habits, repeated surveys and studies have shown that, gradually, over the years, they too become equally prone to the 'big Cs' and all those other Western diseases.

It looks as if it must be something we are eating. Or not eating . . .

15

Thou shalt

Perhaps the main reason why we British are not particularly enthusiastic about positive health maintenance is that sensible medical advice on the subject is mainly concerned with telling us not to do things.

Not doing things is, in general, considerably more difficult than actually doing things. And much more dreary. We are wisely told not to smoke, not to drink much alcohol, not to eat all that sugar or salt or fat. All good advice, but all a matter of 'thou shalt not'.

Until recently, the only medically based 'thou shalt' advice was on the subject of exercise. Thou certainly shouldst do that. The benefits in weight control are obvious, the benefits in physical health undoubted, and the benefits even in mental health becoming increasingly apparent. Physical exercise is becoming known as a valuable tool in treating depression, and if you find that hard to believe just try forcing yourself into a vigorous half hour's sport, jogging or even just a brisk walk next time you feel low, and note the lift in your mood afterwards.

But, exercise apart, the medical profession has been mainly concerned with telling us not to do things, rather than to do things, and banning things rather than advocating them.

It takes a relatively modest amount of scientific evidence to have a substance banned. There are many people, for instance, leading experts among them, who would argue that cyclamates, a useful calorie-free substitute for sugar, were banned on somewhat flimsy evidence involving massive overdosing of animals. Many natural foods we have happily consumed for centuries would never be allowed to be sold in the shops today if they were subject to the same tests as modern drugs and edible substances. This caution obviously arises from the need to minimize the risk of long-term side-effects caused by seemingly innocent new substances.

Conversely, it takes a quite massive amount of scientific evidence to have a substance positively recommended for health. The general attitude of the medical profession is to be highly sceptical, question the benefits, divide into camps and argue bitterly among themselves, and continue scientific testing, surveying and debating for years before becoming convinced.

So when a large body of medical opinion is convinced of the positive benefits of any substance you too can be sure that the evidence must be pretty . . . well, convincing!

This is so of dietary fibre. Today, the medical establishment, in both Britain and America, is of the opinion that dietary fibre is of value in protecting us from the diseases of modern Western civilization. Any list of nutritional recommendations from any eminent medical organization in the Western world will consist of an 'Eat less of these' list (fats, sugar, salt, calories) and a single 'Eat more of this' item. The foods which we are advised to eat in greater quantities are those supplying dietary fibre.

It seems strange that this great surge of medical interest in dietary fibre should have occurred only in the past decade. For very much longer nutritionists have been delving into the values and virtues of vitamins, minerals and the proteins necessary for growth and repair of body tissue. But dietary fibre provides nothing of use in this way. It can be viewed simply as the packaging that encloses these goodies – and who gets excited about the packaging of anything, once it has performed its function of delivering and protecting the goods? Perhaps this was why its importance was overlooked.

When it became known that people in many undeveloped countries remained free of the major killer diseases of Western civilization, it was obvious that medical research into these illnesses should start by delving into the question of what these people were doing, or not doing. One of the things they were doing, it transpires, involves one of man's most private functions – emptying the bowels. Medical friends have told us that one very eminent medical researcher grows so enthusiastic when he shows colour slides of stools excreted by rural Africans that comments like 'Look – aren't they beautiful' fly from his lips during his lecture. Beauty is in the eye of the beholder, of course, and what he is seeing in his mind's eye, after years of study into world-wide distribution of disease in relation to diet, is the stool of someone unlikely to die from cancer of the bowel.

Third World communities who remain free of our degenerative diseases have been found to live on diets which contain a much higher percentage of carbohydrate than ours – carbohydrate obtained from cereals which have not been stripped of their dietary fibre, fibre-rich vegetables (potatoes and other root vegetables), legumes and fruits. The rural African or Asian, living on a diet like this, moves his bowels in a way which can only fill the constipated Western world with envy. Effortlessly, and daily, he evacuates nearly one pound in weight of soft stool – the kind of stool which overwhelms our medical expert with its beauty. In striking contrast the Westerner passes only a quarter of that weight in much firmer, harder stool daily . . . and often not daily . . . and often only with difficulty.

The transit time – the time taken for the food we put into our mouths to pass along the whole of the intestinal tract until the residue is excreted as stools – has also been found to differ enormously between us and them.

In rural Third World communities the average transit time is one and a half days; in Western countries it is about three days in young healthy adults; among the elderly it is often over two weeks.

But does this matter? Only a few years ago, in their efforts to quell the excessive and unhealthy use of laxatives, many doctors were insisting that it did not matter. 'Go when the good Lord moves you,' was the general attitude. 'Some people will move their bowels every day, others only once a week . . . just do what comes naturally.'

We know, from personal experience, that the British nanny and school matron were never really convinced by this argument. It was their view, and that of many an old-fashioned Mum, that the good Lord required a regular daily bowel movement. Come back matron, all is forgiven. It seems that he does. But not by straining, or discipline, or the use of laxatives. When food is eaten in the way that the good Lord grew it, this daily task is accomplished effortlessly and even joyfully.

It is strange how attitudes have come the full circle. People used to have an instinctive feeling that all that waste matter hanging around inside them could not be doing them any good. Hence the popularity, at one time, of some strange practices like collonic irrigation – and the excessive use of laxatives, which was, and still is, condemned on medical grounds. Then, because of these questionable and unnatural methods, doctors began to insist that 'regularity' did not really matter.

Now modern research clearly indicates that a good speedy transit time and daily effortless evacuation of soft stool is indeed a vital protective factor in maintaining our health.

Dietary fibre is the substance which makes the waste matter from the food we eat pass through us and out of us at the desirable, speedy, natural rate. This is one of the main reasons why it is now considered to be such an important protective factor in saving us from diseases of the bowel, like cancer.

Before you continue to discard 'the packaging' with Christmas morning abandon, eating those refined carbohydrate foods, read in the next chapter about the links that are emerging between dietary fibre – or the lack of it – and so many of our Western degenerative diseases and complaints.

16

Major illnesses linked with lack of fibre

In this chapter you will read about the links between intake of dietary fibre and the major Western degenerative diseases – links which connect the factors prevalent in those who fall victim to those illnesses, and in those who do not.

Most people are aware, for instance, that a major link between those who suffer heart attacks is that they tend to have a high level of cholesterol in the blood. This does not necessarily mean that the cholesterol is the cause, or certainly not the sole cause, of heart attacks. But the established association would clearly indicate, at this stage of research, that it isn't a good idea to have too much in your blood.

A diet rich in fibre tends also to be low in fat content because carbohydrate foods provide many of the calories. So these two nutritional factors go together in societies free of our Western ailments – and also in the F-Plan diet.

The F-Plan is a low-fat, low-cholesterol diet, as well as being a high-fibre diet. So it is also the diet to choose if you have sensibly taken to heart the well-established benefits of reducing fat intake.

Dietary fibre and cancer of the colon

There is a vast variation in the incidence of cancer of the colon in different countries throughout the world. In America it is the most common fatal form of cancer, in Britain it is second only to cancer of the lung. In many undeveloped countries it is virtually unknown. There is little doubt, in the view of even the most conservative members of the medical establishment, that the cause of large bowel cancer is environmental and that the factors involved are related to economic development. The greater the degree of economic development, the greater the incidence of cancer of the colon.

No other form of cancer has been found to be more closely related to the Western way of life – and the Western way of eating. Research is showing that diets which appear perfectly all right in other respects may lead to processes occurring within the gut that could increase the production or the concentration of cancer-inducing substances – carcinogens.

There are various ways in which fibre-depleted foods are now thought to be linked with cancer of the large bowel. Firstly, the small stools of Western man will have a higher concentration of these cancer-inducing substances than the large diluted stools of the fibre eater. The slow transit rate of fibre-depleted diets is also thought to encourage the formation of these potentially dangerous substances within the body – and to leave them in contact with the gut for too long.

In short, the basic instinct which seemed to tell many people that they needed a good 'clean out', and that nasty things could happen while waste matter lingered around in the body, seems to have been largely correct. It was only the unnatural methods they used in order to combat the problem which were wrong.

Bowel cancer is invariably rare in communities passing large stools, and stool volume is always small in communities with a high frequency of bowel cancer. It is dietary fibre, of course, which affects this stool volume. In rural Finns, for example, who consume a relatively high fibre diet, cancer of the colon is rare. They have been found to eat about twice as much dietary fibre as New Yorkers, among whom this form of cancer is rife.

Perhaps the most compelling evidence of all comes from studies of people who have moved from one country to another – Japanese who have emigrated to California, for instance – and adopted Western diets. Large bowel cancer is uncommon among Japanese eating their traditional diet, but it was found that, within a generation, Japanese eating the American way had developed a risk of large bowel cancer equal to that of Americans. This strongly endorses the 'it-must-be-something-we-eat' theory as against the theory of the genetic susceptibility to certain diseases of different races.

The strong dietary links emerge from studies of communities with high and low incidence of this form of cancer. Those at high risk are eating a lot of fat and very little dietary fibre. Those at low risk are doing just the reverse. All the evidence available clearly suggests that excessive fat in the diet increases the risk of developing large bowel cancer and that fibre provides protection against it. The Royal College of Physicians has gone on record as stating that 'there are reasonable grounds for the statement that, in genetically susceptible persons, large bowel cancer could be favoured by a fibre-depleted diet'. Though they add, of course, that other explanations for the prevalence of this cancer in Westernized countries are possible.

This statement, from such a conservative and distinguished authority, certainly puts the idea that dietary fibre is beneficial well beyond the 'crank threshold'. For all sensible people it would clearly suggest that more thought should be given to the fibre content not only of their own diets, but of those of their children.

Dietary fibre and coronary heart disease

Coronary heart disease is essentially a modern Western disease and was rare, even in Western countries, until after the First World War. Today it is the commonest cause of death in the West. It remains almost unknown among rural Africans and is uncommon in most rural communities in Asia. The evidence suggests that a variety of factors in our modern Western environment – cigarette smoking, diet, sedentary living, soft water, stress – may be involved. In our diets, emphasis has for many years been laid on the intake of saturated fat as the major danger factor, but this is certainly not the whole explanation.

When a project researching into the cause of this disease carefully examined a group of men in London, recording their way of life and following their subsequent history for twenty years or until they died, the strongest risk factor for coronary heart disease was found to be smoking and the strongest protective factor the intake of cereal fibre.

The dietary fibre connection is not in any way as clear and direct as it is in the evidence concerning cancer of the colon. But what evidence has emerged about dietary fibre certainly puts it among the 'good guys', helping to protect us from heart disease, as opposed to the 'bad guys' like animal fats and smoking.

The 'good guys' so far seem to consist of a team of two.

Bad guys   (factors which are thought possibly to increase risk of coronary heart disease)

Being overweight; smoking; suffering from stress; eating too much animal fat; eating too much cholesterol-containing food (like eggs); eating too much salt; eating too much refined sugar; sedentary living.

Good guys   (factors which are thought to help prevent coronary heart disease)
Taking sufficient prolonged exercise; consuming sufficient dietary fibre.

One of the reasons for the beneficial effect of dietary fibre is that it reduces the absorption of cholesterol – but there are other ways, too, in which it would appear to perform useful functions in keeping the heart healthy.

The evidence in favour of dietary fibre as a preventative measure in heart disease is not strong enough to be conclusive at this stage, but is certainly strong enough to be thought-provoking.

Diverticular disease of the colon

This is another of those modern Western diseases that seems to have mushroomed up from nowhere over the past fifty years. But only over here – not over there. It is almost unknown in Africa and Asia, while in the West, from being relatively rare as recently as the 1920s, it has now become the commonest disorder of the large intestine. It is said to be present, although usually without symptoms, in one in ten people over the age of forty, and in one in three over the age of sixty.

Constipation is now recognized as the underlying cause of this disease – and fibre-depleted diets are recognized as the major cause of constipation.

It is the effort and pressure which the bowel-wall muscle has to exert in propelling onward the firm faeces produced by a Western diet (rather than the soft and voluminous matter produced by fibre-rich diets) which has been found to be the cause of this illness.

In relation to diverticular disease the beneficial role of dietary fibre is very clear. Today a fibre-rich diet, often including bran, is not only advocated as a preventative measure: it is also widely used in the treatment of this disease. Since the advent of treatment with bran, fewer patients have required surgery for the complications of diverticular disease.

Dietary fibre and diabetes

Having read earlier about the 'rebound hunger' factor involved in diets consisting of large quantities of refined carbohydrate foods, you will already have gained some clue to the role that dietary fibre can play in the prevention and control of adult-onset diabetes, particularly common among overweight people.

In Western populations a fairly large proportion of people develop difficulty in utilizing carbohydrates in their diets during middle age. This difficulty is caused by a fault in the insulin production of the body. Insulin, as we have already explained, is necessary to control excess blood sugar. If blood-sugar level rises too high then sugar also appears in the urine and the person may be regarded as a diabetic.

As well as diabetics, there is a borderline group of people who are better classified as having 'impaired glucose tolerance' rather than being frank diabetics. Though only a small proportion go on to develop diabetes, these subjects have an increased risk of death from cardio-vascular disease.

As we have explained earlier in the book, insulin response to the carbohydrate foods we eat varies with the speed of absorption of the carbohydrate. Any dietary factor which delays the absorption of carbo-hydrate may be regarded as beneficial – and here, once again, is where dietary fibre appears in a valuable preventative and protective role. Carbohydrate foods rich in fibre are absorbed more slowly than those from which the fibre has been stripped.

It looks as if the adult-onset type of diabetes is most likely to appear among those who eat refined low-fibre foods. Again, it has been found to be uncommon among those living on traditional unprocessed foods. In the United States, it has been found that a diet very rich in unrefined high-fibre starch has caused remission of the disease in 85 per cent of the adult-onset diabetic patients on which it has been tested.

This change of diet should not, of course, be attempted by diabetics except under medical supervision, and so far no juvenile diabetics have been treated successfully using this type of diet. However, more doctors are beginning to recommend more unrefined high-fibre starch foods in diabetic diets and once again it seems as if fibre points the way to a healthier future.

17

Little things that mean a lot

It is not the purpose of this book to provide a complete medical directory of all the illnesses that are attributed, at least in some measure, to lack of natural fibre in the Western diet. We simply want to emphasize that the medical indications for the need of more of this substance in our diets are strong and impressive. This is not simply a passing fad.

If you have not been impressed by the very positive connection between a lack of dietary fibre and the incidence of cancer of the colon, and the possible connections between fibre and heart disease, you are unlikely to rush off for a wholemeal loaf in order to prevent appendicitis or gall stones, just two of the other ailments being associated with our fibre-depleted modern diets.

However, little things which affect our vanity often influence us more strongly than major things which could affect our health. Possibly because we don't take an 'oh, that couldn't possibly happen to me' attitude to the former.

In our view, the advertising award of the decade should go to the brain who thought up the series of anti-smoking television adverts which did not even mention lung cancer, but drew attention to the fact that smoking gives you bad breath. Well done, sir! Possibly an HM government warning about bad breath would be more effective than the present slogan.

Certainly, the enlightened medical-research award of the future should go to any researcher who has the wit to do further investigation into the connection between smoking and the complexion. So far, one survey has clearly suggested that smoking makes the skin wrinkle sooner, but research seems to have stopped there. How amazing. How remarkable that it doesn't seem to have occurred to the medical profession that earlier wrinkles would be a motivation without parallel in encouraging the female half of the population (at least) to abandon the nasty habit.

However, it has occurred to us that to mention some of the unglamorous little things that can happen to you if you don't might be highly effective in getting you to eat up your dietary fibre.

For starters – varicose veins

We all know what varicose veins look like. Those who haven't got them certainly don't want them, and those who have them already certainly don't want them to get worse.

Oddly enough, the initial cause of varicose veins is not fully understood, but there are some eminent medical researchers, like Dr Denis Burkitt, who believe that the major cause of varicose veins is increased abdominal pressure caused by straining to pass small, firm, Western-style stools. Hurry off for the bran.

For male readers – haemorrhoids

There is simply no sex appeal in a haemorrhoid. Surprisingly little sympathy too – considering the discomfort haemorrhoids can cause. Wary sufferers will have learned to suffer silently lest they raise stifled giggles rather than sympathy.

Considering the nature of the ailment it will come as no surprise that one of the major causes is thought to be constipation and, again, the straining involved in evacuating a hard faecal mass. In recent years it has been found that a high proportion of patients suffering from piles require no further treatment once they have switched to a high-fibre diet and as a result pass soft stools that can be evacuated with minimal straining.

For the kiddiwinks – bad teeth

Most children are probably sick of hearing about bad teeth, but the guardians of their dental health will be interested to note that the Royal College of Physicians quite firmly advocates a fibre-rich diet which 'encourages mastication' for the good of the teeth. Those teeth were made to chew with. If they are not used in the way nature intended they become more subject to dental disease and caries; chewing fibre-rich foods helps to keep the teeth cleaner and free of plaque in a variety of different ways.

After years of medical doubt it is at last safe to say with conviction that an apple a day – along with the other fibre-rich foods you will eat on the F-Plan – does indeed keep the doctor away. And also the dentist.

18

The ever-after fibre factor

Probably the most depressing words that have ever been pronounced about any slimming diet are those enthusiastic phrases from well-meaning medics on the lines of 'This is a diet that you can follow for the rest of your life.' Normal human beings will discard all thought of even starting any such diet – instantly! Who on earth wants to think of following a slimming diet for ever.

Do not throw this book away. We are most positively not going to say anything like that. What we are going to say is simply that the parts of this diet which are easy and effortless and even enjoyable to you will become part of your normal eating in the future.

Quite probably you simply didn't realize that peas and beans and sweetcorn are such valuable vegetables, and you will now continue to eat them rather more frequently because you like them anyway.

Having tried bran flakes you might well find that you like them just as much as ordinary cornflakes. There isn't much difference in the flavour. And if you find that sprinkling on just a little bran in no way detracts from your bowl of breakfast cereal, then you will be tempted to continue to do so.

Preferences between wholemeal bread and white bread are largely a matter of habit. Having become accustomed to wholemeal bread during your F-Plan slimming programme you might well find that, by the time you have got slim, you have actually grown to prefer it.

Once you have shed your surplus weight you will be able to increase your food intake, and on a normal quota of calories it isn't at all difficult to increase your dietary fibre intake to 40g a day just by becoming aware of the fibre-rich foods – as you will during the following weeks. It is considered that something in the region of 40g daily should be quite sufficient to protect your health in all the ways which have been described, and to make it much easier for you to control your weight in the future.

If you are a parent it is almost certain that your increased awareness of the value of dietary fibre will start to influence the foods you provide for the family – and thus their habits and preferences in the future.

The major Western degenerative diseases don't happen in an instant – like infective diseases – but appear to creep up on us slowly as a result of years and years of bad eating.

Although you will never know it, it could be that the slimming diet you are about to embark on will prevent your own children from suffering from cancer of the colon, forty years from now. Quite a bonus, when you think of it.

19

The F-Plan diet rules

Here are the essential rules to follow in order to shed your surplus weight on the F-Plan diet:

1. Determine your total daily calorie intake at a minimum figure of 850 and a maximum of 1,500. Read Chapter 9 for guidance on your ideal dieting calorie total.

2. Choose your foods from the charts to ensure a daily intake of more than 30g of dietary fibre. Between 35g and 50g is the F-Plan recommendation, but this could be lowered a little by those on very low-calorie, short-term slimming programmes.

3. Have half a pint of skimmed milk each day. This supplies 100 calories, which must be subtracted from your daily total.

4. Apart from milk, drink only those drinks which are negligible in calorie content. These are listed in Chapter 11. (If you find it difficult to diet without enjoying a moderate amount of alcohol, refer to Chapter 11 for advice and guidance on how this can be made possible.)

5. Have two whole fresh fruits each day, either an apple or a pear, and an orange. No need to weigh these fruits; day-to-day variations will tend to balance out the calorie and fibre content. Subtract another 100 calories from your daily total for this fruit and add 5g to your fibre total.

6. Eat the daily quantity of Fibre-Filler – the ingredients and amounts are given on page 65. Divide this into two portions, each mixed with milk from the daily half pint; have one of these for breakfast and the other at any time later in the day. To account for the Fibre-Filler, subtract 200 from your daily calorie total and add 15g to your daily fibre total. Have one of the breakfasts listed on pages 205 and 206 *only* if you don't have Fibre-Filler.

7. To get maximum benefit in making your diet easy, speed and healthy, obtain your dietary fibre from a wide range of cereal, fruit and vegetable foods – rather than seeking to make up the total from just one or two very fibre-rich foods.

8. Choose freely from the calorie- and fibre-counted meals on the

following pages to make up the remainder of your daily calorie and fibre total. As you get used to the F-Plan method you will probably want to plan your own high-fibre meals and can do so easily with the calorie and fibre charts at the back of the book.

This is all much more simple than it might seem from the previous, necessarily precise, rules. It works out this way. Your daily milk, two pieces of fresh fruit and portion of Fibre-Filler add up to a total of 400 calories and 20g of fibre. Subtract these calories from your total for the day and make up the rest from other meals. Also, make up your additional 15g or more of dietary fibre from the meals – so that your total daily intake of dietary fibre is, ideally, between 35g and 50g.

If you are dieting on 850 calories a day, choose meals adding up to 450 calories a day.

If you are dieting on 1,000 calories a day, choose meals adding up to 600 calories a day.

If you are dieting on 1,250 calories a day, choose meals adding up to 850 calories a day.

If you are dieting on 1,500 calories a day, you can choose meals adding up to 1,100 calories a day.

When you eat and how often you eat is entirely up to you as long as you keep to the correct calorie total and aim for the right fibre total. Some people prefer to save a large proportion of their calories for a big evening meal, and others prefer to eat small meals more frequently. 'Do your own thing' is excellent advice in dieting – because 'your own thing' tends to be the easiest thing for you, and the diet method that is easy is the one you will succeed in keeping to.

The F-Plan recipes, meal suggestions and charts on the following pages give you plenty of scope both for doing your own thing and eating your own thing, whether it is something as simple as beans on toast or a sandwich, or something considerably more adventurous.

A word about your weight loss

From the day you start F-Plan dieting you will start shedding surplus fat. But, because you are eating fibre-rich food, it may be three or four days before the loss of that fat becomes apparent on the scales.

The reason is simply a minor fluctuation in the fluid content of your body. Remember, fibre-rich food holds extra water, so two or three extra pounds of liquid retained inside you can easily obscure the same quantity of lost fat. Be patient. By the end of the first week's dieting the scales will start to reveal the true story of your excellent rate of weight loss, and from then on it will be downhill all the way to your ideal weight!

One little 'running yourself in' problem may occur as you switch to this healthier pattern of eating. Those who have become used to low-fibre food may suffer from a little flatulence for the first week or two. This problem should soon resolve itself as you adjust to the diet. If you do find this a particular problem during the early stages of F-Plan dieting, concentrate on the meals which do not have a high content of peas and beans until you have become accustomed to high-fibre eating.

Important health note

If you are overweight but are otherwise in sound health, it would be unrealistic to ask you to get your doctor's permission to diet. However, if you suffer from any health complications it would be wise to tell your doctor that you are planning to follow a high-fibre, low-calorie diet, and to ask his advice. Happily, apart from patients with high-grade obstruction within the alimentary tract, or with coeliac disease, dietary fibre in its natural state in food has not been shown to cause or exacerbate any human disease in the Western population. Its effect, as you will have read earlier in the book, is to protect you from ill-health rather than cause it.

The F-Plan meals

THE F-PLAN MEALS

The quantities for most of the meals on the following pages are given for a single portion. Experience shows that dieters very often prefer to eat alone rather than at the family table – contrary to the exhortation 'make this for the family too' beloved by diet experts.

As you read of the great virtues of dietary fibre in the prevention of illness you will almost certainly want to introduce more fibre in the general family diet. But it is generally more helpful to give meals for slimmers in single portions – and it is very easy to multiply up the quantities, of course.

Where a fairly lengthy list of ingredients is involved, and a little more time, *and where the recipe will freeze*, we have given recipes for four portions. This is to save you time in the kitchen, which is a very hazard-filled area for slimmers. The less time spent there, the better.

When you make these dishes, or other obviously easily freezable recipes which you particularly like, it is a good idea to cook several portions at one time and then divide them into individual portions and store them in the freezer in bags. A freezer well stocked with little bags, each containing a prepared calorie-counted and fibre-counted meal, provides excellent protection against temptation to break your diet simply because you haven't had time to shop for the right foods.

All these meals are grouped into sections based on the fibre-rich food which forms the main ingredient of the meal. In each section the individual meals are listed in rising order of calorie value. You will find the lowest calorie meals at the start of the section, the highest at the end. Any four-portion recipes are listed at the end of the appropriate section.

We have rounded off calorie values of meals to make it easy for you to add together your 450–1,000 calories allowed for the day (in addition to your 400 from Fibre-Filler, fruit and milk); we have also rounded off metric ingredient figures for easy measuring. The amount of fibre provided by each meal is given (in grams) beside the calorie count. Again we have done a little rounding off of figures to avoid decimal points.

The meals themselves are designed to cater for all tastes. They include some very simple meals as well as some more imaginative dishes. We believe you will find it quite difficult not to find a large number of meals which appeal to you, because no less than six cookery experts have combined their various tastes and talents to provide this selection of low-calorie, high-fibre meals.

The desserts can be consumed with an utterly clear conscience when you have calories to spare in your daily allowance. They provide you with fibre and healthy nutrients in place of the usual surplus calories, tooth decay and guilt.

On pages 206–211 we give some sample ready-planned daily menus made up from these meals, to show you how easy it is to keep to your preferred eating pattern and daily dieting calorie allowance.

Note. Where quantities are measured in spoonfuls we mean a *level* spoonful unless otherwise indicated. We use the standard teaspoon of 5 ml, the standard tablespoon of 15 ml capacity.

BREAKFASTS

F-Plan dieters should ideally breakfast on a portion of their Fibre-Filler. These fibre-rich breakfasts are only for those who want an alternative. Milk should be used from the daily allowance. For this reason it is not included in the calorie total.

PUFFED WHEAT PLUS BRAN

Calories 100; Fibre 6g

½oz (15g) Puffed Wheat
¼oz (7g) bran
½oz (15g) sultanas

ALL BRAN AND SULTANAS

Calories 150; Fibre 12g

1½oz (40g) All Bran or Bran Buds
½oz (15g) sultanas

ALLINSON'S HONEY BRAN

Calories 150; Fibre 9g

1½oz (40g) Allinson's Honey Bran
½oz (15g) sultanas

PREWETT'S BRAN MUESLI

Calories 175; Fibre 12g

2oz (55g) serving

ENERGEN BRAN CRUNCH

Calories 200; Fibre 7g

1½oz (40g) Energen Bran Crunch
½oz (15g) sultanas

BRAN FLAKES PLUS BRAN

Calories 200; Fibre 8g

1½oz (40g) Bran Flakes
½oz (15g) sultanas
¼oz (7g) bran

BAKED JACKET POTATO MEALS

All the meals listed in this section begin with a 7oz (200g) raw-weight potato. The potato is first baked in its jacket and then it can be used in one of the variety of meals which follow, either as an accompaniment to other foods (for example, baked chicken joint and sweetcorn) or stuffed (for example, with cheese and pickle). The baked jacket potato, on its own, provides 175 calories and at least 5g fibre – remember to eat the jacket too, because this is a good source of dietary fibre.

Baked potato served on its own screams out for butter or soured cream to moisten it, but since these are high-calorie foods, two low-calorie dressings which will moisten and add flavour have been given with the basic recipe. If these do not appear in your baked jacket potato meal and you wish to use one of them on your potato, just add the calorie value to your daily calorie total. Where they are included in a meal, the calorie value has also been included.

To complete one of the stuffed baked jacket potato meals you might like to add a salad, so we have included two low-calorie salads after the basic recipe, on page 105; just add the calorie value and fibre content to your daily totals.

BAKED JACKET POTATO – BASIC RECIPE

Calories 175; Fibre 5g

7oz (200g) potato

Scrub the potato well, then bake by one of the following methods:
1. Place the potato in the centre of a moderately hot oven (400°F, 200°C, gas 6) for 45 minutes or until soft when pinched.
2. Place the potato in a pan of water, bring to the boil, then simmer gently for 20 minutes. Drain, then place the potato in a moderate oven (375°F, 190°C, gas 5) for 10–15 minutes to crisp the skin.
3. Prick well all over and cook in a microwave oven on full power for 4 minutes, turning over after 2 minutes.
Serve the baked potato as a vegetable accompaniment, with one of the dressings listed below to moisten, if preferred, or serve in one of the following meals.

TOMATO YOGURT DRESSING

Calories 25

2 tablespoons low-fat natural yogurt
1 teaspoon tomato purée
salt and pepper
a dash of Worcestershire sauce (optional)

Mix the yogurt with the tomato purée until evenly blended. Season to taste with salt and pepper and add Worcestershire sauce, if liked. Spoon over the cut surface of a baked jacket potato.

CHEESY POTATO DRESSING

Calories 25

1 tablespoon cottage cheese with chives
2 tablespoons Waistline Oil-Free French Dressing

Beat the cottage cheese and dressing together until well blended. Spoon over the cut surface of a baked jacket potato.

ITALIAN COD WITH BAKED JACKET POTATO

Calories 300; Fibre 9g

7oz (200g) potato
4oz (115g) frozen cod steak
8oz (225g) canned tomatoes
1oz (25g) chopped onion
1oz (25g) chopped green pepper
pinch dried oregano or $\frac{1}{2}$ teaspoon chopped fresh oregano
1 tablespoon bran
salt and freshly ground black pepper

Scrub the potato and bake in a moderately hot oven for 15 minutes. Meanwhile place the frozen cod steak in a small ovenproof dish or casserole. Chop the canned tomatoes and mix with the juice, onion, green pepper, oregano, bran and seasoning to taste. Spoon over the fish. Cover and bake with the potato for another 30 minutes. Serve with the baked potato.

COTTAGE CHEESE SALAD WITH BAKED JACKET POTATO

Calories 350; Fibre 8g

7oz (200g) potato
4oz (115g) cottage cheese (natural or with chives or onion and peppers)
1 walnut half
a few lettuce leaves
a small bunch watercress (about 1oz, 25g)
1 small onion, cut into rings
1 small orange, segmented and membranes removed

Prepare and bake the potato (see p. 99). Serve with the cottage cheese garnished with the walnut half and with a salad prepared from the lettuce, watercress, onion rings and orange segments.

GRILLED BACON STEAK WITH BAKED JACKET POTATO AND BAKED BEANS

Calories 375; Fibre 8g

7oz (200g) potato
3½oz (100g) bacon steak
4oz (115g) baked beans

Prepare and bake the potato (see p. 99). Grill the bacon steak without added fat until cooked through. Heat the baked beans. Serve the baked potato with the grilled bacon steak and baked beans.

HAM AND COLESLAW SALAD WITH BAKED JACKET POTATO

Calories 375; Fibre 11g

7oz (200g) potato
2oz (55g) sliced lean boiled ham
3oz (85g) firm white cabbage, shredded
2oz (55g) carrot, grated
2 sticks celery, finely chopped
1 tablespoon chopped fresh parsley
1 tablespoon Waistline Oil-Free French Dressing
1 tablespoon low-fat natural yogurt
1 portion cheesy potato dressing (p. 100)
½ carton mustard and cress

Prepare and bake the potato (see p. 99). Trim off and discard any fat on the ham. Mix the cabbage, carrot, celery and parsley together in a bowl. Blend the French dressing and yogurt together and stir into the vegetable mixture. Divide the coleslaw between the two slices of ham and roll the ham around it. Serve the ham and coleslaw rolls with the baked jacket potato topped with cheesy potato dressing and garnish with the mustard and cress.

PILCHARD SALAD WITH BAKED JACKET POTATO

Calories 375; Fibre 13g

7oz (200g) potato
1 portion cheesy potato dressing (p. 100)
4oz (115g) canned pilchards
2 sticks celery, chopped
2oz (55g) carrot, grated
2oz (55g) fresh garden peas or thawed frozen peas
1 tablespoon Waistline Oil-Free French Dressing
a few lettuce leaves

Prepare and bake the potato (see p. 99). Mix the celery, carrot, peas and French dressing together. Place the lettuce leaves on the plate with the pilchards and baked potato and pile the celery salad on top. Serve with the cheesy dressing.

BAKED CHICKEN, JACKET POTATO AND SWEETCORN

Calories 400; Fibre 8g

7oz (200g) potato
8oz (225g) chicken joint
2oz (55g) frozen or canned sweetcorn kernels
1 portion tomato yogurt dressing (p. 100)
sprigs of watercress (optional)

Scrub the potato. Wrap the chicken joint in foil and bake with the potato in the oven at 400°F (200°C, gas 6) for 30 minutes. Open the foil so that the chicken can continue to cook uncovered. Bake for a further 10 minutes. Meanwhile cook the sweetcorn as directed on the packet and drain. Remove and discard the skin from the chicken. Split the baked potato in half lengthways, and top with the tomato yogurt dressing. Serve the chicken with the baked potato and sweetcorn, and a few sprigs of watercress, if liked.

GRILLED BEEFBURGERS WITH BAKED JACKET POTATO AND PEAS

Calories 400; Fibre 10g

7oz (200g) potato
2 × 2oz (55g) frozen beefburgers
2oz (55g) frozen peas
1 portion tomato yogurt dressing (p. 100)

Prepare and bake the potato (see p. 99). Grill the beefburgers well on both sides so that much of the fat drips away. Cook the peas as directed. Serve the jacket potato with the tomato yogurt dressing, beefburgers and peas.

GRILLED LAMB CHOP WITH BAKED JACKET POTATO, SPROUTS AND CARROTS

Calories 450; Fibre 10g

7oz (200g) potato
4oz (115g) lamb loin chop
3oz (85g) Brussels sprouts
2oz (55g) carrots, sliced
1 portion cheesy potato dressing (p. 100)
2 teaspoons mint sauce

Prepare and bake the potato (see p. 99). Grill the lamb chop without added fat until cooked through. Boil the Brussels sprouts and carrots until just tender, then drain. Split the baked potato and top with the cheesy dressing. Serve with the lamb chop, mint sauce, Brussels sprouts and carrots.

LIVER CASSEROLE WITH BAKED JACKET POTATO

Calories 450; Fibre 12g

7oz (200g) potato
4oz (115g) lamb's liver, sliced
salt and freshly ground pepper
2oz (55g) onion, sliced
1 stick celery, chopped
8oz (225g) canned tomatoes
1 teaspoon Worcestershire sauce
2oz (55g) Brussels sprouts

Scrub the potato. Arrange the lamb's liver in the bottom of an oven-proof dish and season to taste. Put the onion rings and celery on top. Chop the canned tomatoes and mix with the Worcestershire sauce. Spoon with the tomato juices over the liver and vegetables. Season with salt and pepper. Cover and cook with the potato in the oven at 375°F (190°C, gas 5) for 45 minutes or until the potato is soft and the liver cooked. Boil the Brussels sprouts and serve with the casserole and baked potato.

STUFFED BAKED JACKET POTATO MEALS – BASIC RECIPE

Calories 175; Fibre 5g

7oz (200g) baked jacket potato (p. 99)

Cut the potato in half lengthwise and scoop out some of the flesh. Mix with one of the fillings described in the meals below and pile back into the potato jacket. Heat through in the oven for 5–10 minutes, if necessary.

Salad vegetables make an ideal accompaniment to these stuffed baked potatoes. The following two simple salads may be added to any of the stuffed baked potato meals. (Remember to add the calories to your total.)

MIXED SALAD

Calories 25; Fibre 2g

a few lettuce leaves
a 1in (2·5cm) piece cucumber, sliced
1 medium tomato, sliced
2 spring onions, chopped, or ½oz (15g) onion rings
1oz (25g) green or red pepper, sliced and chopped
1 tablespoon Waistline Oil-Free French Dressing

Arrange the salad vegetables in a bowl and toss with the dressing.

COLESLAW

Calories 50; Fibre 4g

3oz (85g) white cabbage, shredded
2oz (55g) carrot, grated
1 tablespoon Heinz Slimway Low-Calorie Salad Dressing

Mix the cabbage, carrot and salad dressing together until thoroughly blended.

SCRAMBLED EGG AND TOMATO STUFFED JACKET POTATO

Calories 275; Fibre 6g

1 egg, size 3
2 tablespoons skimmed milk
salt and pepper
1 medium tomato, chopped
7oz (200g) baked jacket potato (p. 99)
sprigs of parsley

Scramble the egg with the skimmed milk and seasoning in a non-stick pan. Stir in the tomato. Mash the potato flesh and mix with the scrambled egg. Pile into the potato jacket and serve garnished with sprigs of parsley.

FISH AND SWEETCORN STUFFED JACKET POTATO

Calories 275; Fibre 7g

3¼oz (92g) pack frozen coley or cod steak
1oz (25g) canned sweetcorn kernels
7oz (200g) baked jacket potato (p. 99)
1 tablespoon tomato sauce

Poach the frozen fish steak in a little water until cooked through. Drain and flake the fish. Cook the sweetcorn and drain. Prepare the stuffed potato using the flaked fish, sweetcorn and tomato sauce. Heat through in the oven if necessary.

SAUSAGE AND MUSTARD PICKLE STUFFED JACKET POTATO

Calories 300; Fibre 5g

2 beef chipolata sausages
1 tablespoon mustard pickle
7oz (200g) baked jacket potato (p. 99)
2 sprigs watercress

Grill the sausages well. Slice into small pieces and mix with the mustard pickle and the flesh from the potato. Pile into the potato jacket and heat through if required. Serve garnished with watercress.

CHICKEN AND PEPPERS STUFFED JACKET POTATO

Calories 300; Fibre 6g

2oz (55g) roast chicken
1oz (25g) green pepper, chopped
1oz (25g) red pepper, chopped
1 tablespoon low-calorie salad dressing
7oz (200g) baked jacket potato (p. 99)
2 tablespoons skimmed milk
salt and pepper

Remove and discard any skin from the chicken; chop the meat. Mix with the chopped peppers and salad dressing. Mash the potato flesh with the skimmed milk and seasoning to taste, then mix with the chicken and peppers. Pile back into the potato jacket. Reheat in the oven.

CHEESE AND PICKLE STUFFED JACKET POTATO WITH SALAD

Calories 300; Fibre 8g

7oz (200g) baked jacket potato (p. 99)
2oz (55g) natural cottage cheese
1 rounded tablespoon sweet pickle

Mixed salad
a few lettuce leaves
2oz (55g) sliced green pepper
1 medium tomato, sliced
1oz (25g) watercress
2 spring onions, chopped
1 tablespoon Waistline Oil-Free French Dressing

Prepare the stuffed potato as described on p. 105 using the cottage cheese and pickle to fill. Serve with the mixed salad.

PRAWN, SWEETCORN AND SPRING ONION STUFFED JACKET POTATO

Calories 300; Fibre 9g

2oz (55g) fresh or frozen prawns
7oz (200g) baked jacket potato (p. 99)
1oz (25g) canned sweetcorn kernels
2 spring onions, chopped
1 tablespoon low-calorie salad dressing
2 medium or 1 large tomato, halved and sliced

Thaw the prawns if frozen. Mix the mashed potato flesh with the prawns, sweetcorn, spring onions and salad dressing. Pile back into the potato jacket. Serve garnished with the tomato.

CHEESE AND BAKED BEANS STUFFED JACKET POTATO

Calories 300; Fibre 10g

7oz (200g) baked jacket potato (p. 99)
2oz (55g) baked beans
1oz (25g) Edam cheese, grated
a small bunch of watercress, about 1oz (25g)

Prepare the stuffed potato as described above, using the baked beans and grated cheese to fill. Serve with the watercress.

CHEESY GRILLED JACKET POTATO

Calories 325; Fibre 6g

7oz (200g) baked jacket potato (p. 99)
2 tablespoons skimmed milk
1½oz (40g) Edam cheese, grated
1 medium tomato, chopped
salt and pepper
grated nutmeg

Mix the potato flesh with the remaining ingredients, reserving ½oz (15g) grated cheese. Pile the mixture back into the potato jacket, sprinkle the tops with the remaining grated cheese. Place under a hot grill until the cheese has melted.

HAM, SWEETCORN AND CELERY STUFFED JACKET POTATO

Calories 325; Fibre 8g

7oz (200g) baked jacket potato (p. 99)
2 tablespoons skimmed milk
salt and pepper
2oz (55g) lean cooked ham
1 tablespoon canned sweetcorn kernels
1 stick celery, finely chopped
a few sprigs of watercress

Scoop the flesh out of the potato and mash with the skimmed milk and seasoning to taste. Chop the ham, discarding any fat. Add the ham, sweetcorn and celery to the potato and mix together. Pile back into the jacket and heat through in the oven. Serve garnished with watercress.

CHICKEN LIVERS AND MUSHROOM STUFFED JACKET POTATO

Calories 350; Fibre 7g

4oz (115g) chicken livers, chopped
1oz (25g) mushrooms, sliced
1 tablespoon finely chopped onion
4 tablespoons chicken stock
salt and pepper
a dash of tabasco sauce
7oz (200g) baked jacket potato (p. 99)
2oz (55g) white cabbage, chopped

Place the chicken livers, mushrooms, onion and stock in a small pan. Add the salt and pepper and tabasco sauce. Heat to simmering point, cover and cook gently for 5 minutes. Prepare the stuffed potato as described on p. 105, using the chicken liver mixture to fill. Serve with the chopped cabbage either raw or lightly boiled.

MUSHROOM, EGG AND BACON STUFFED JACKET POTATO

Calories 350; Fibre 7g

1 rasher streaky bacon
3oz (85g) mushrooms
1 egg, size 3
salt and pepper
¼oz (7g) low-fat spread
7oz (200g) baked jacket potato (p. 99)
½ carton mustard and cress

Grill the bacon rasher until crisp, and crumble or chop it. Chop the mushrooms and simmer in a little salted water for 5 minutes, then drain. Beat the egg with salt and pepper and stir in the bacon and mushrooms. Melt the low-fat spread in a small pan and add the egg mixture. Cook over a low heat until the egg is just set. Stir in the potato flesh and pile into the potato jacket. Garnish with the mustard and cress.

SARDINE AND COTTAGE CHEESE STUFFED JACKET POTATO

Calories 350; Fibre 7g

2 sardines canned in tomato sauce
2oz (55g) cottage cheese
7oz (200g) baked jacket potato (p. 99)
1 teaspoon finely chopped onion or chives
1oz (25g) frozen peas, cooked
salt and pepper
sprigs of watercress

Mash the sardines with the cottage cheese and potato flesh. Add the onion or chives, peas and seasoning to taste. Pile into the potato jacket and heat through in the oven. Serve garnished with the watercress.

SAVOURY MINCED BEEF STUFFED JACKET POTATO

Calories 375; Fibre 6g

4oz (115g) raw minced beef
1oz (25g) chopped onion
1oz (25g) grated carrot
1 teaspoon concentrated curry sauce
7oz (200g) baked jacket potato (p. 99)
salt and pepper

Fry the minced beef in a heavy saucepan without added fat until well browned. Drain off and discard the fat. Add the onion, carrot, curry sauce and 4–5 tablespoons water. Heat until boiling, then simmer, covered, for 15 minutes. Cut the potato in two lengthwise, scoop out some of the flesh and mix with the hot minced beef mixture. Season to taste. Pile back into the jackets and serve at once.

PEANUTS AND TOMATO STUFFED JACKET POTATO

Calories 375; Fibre 11g

7oz (200g) baked jacket potato (p. 99)
1oz (25g) salted peanuts
1 large tomato, about 4 oz (115g), chopped
freshly ground pepper
a few sprigs of watercress
3oz (85g) Chinese leaves, shredded
1 tablespoon lemon juice

Mix the potato flesh with the peanuts and chopped tomato and pile into the potato jacket. Season with pepper. Reheat. Garnish with sprigs of watercress. Serve with the Chinese leaves tossed in lemon juice.

COD AND SAUCE STUFFED JACKET POTATO

Calories 400; Fibre 12g

7oz (200g) baked jacket potato (p. 99)
6oz (170g) pack frozen cod in parsley sauce
a sprig of parsley
3oz (85g) frozen peas

Cook the frozen cod in parsley sauce as directed on the packet. Flake the fish into the sauce. Mix the mashed potato flesh with the fish and sauce. Pile into the potato jacket and heat through in the oven. Cook the peas as directed and serve with the stuffed potato.

'SAVOURY CUT' CASSEROLE WITH BAKED JACKET POTATO – TWO SERVINGS

Two portions: 950 calories; 32g fibre
Individual portion: 475 calories; 16g fibre

7oz (200g) potato for jacket baking, per serving
4·97oz (141g) can Farrow Giant Marrowfat Processed Peas
1 small onion, chopped
7oz (198g) can Sainsbury's Sliced Young Carrots
7½oz (213g) can Granose Savoury Cuts

Scrub the potato and bake in a moderately hot oven for 45 minutes or until tender. Cut the savoury cuts into cubes and place in a casserole with all the sauce. Stir in the onion and drained carrots. Cover with a lid or foil and cook near the bottom of the oven with the potato. Add the drained peas 10 minutes before the end of cooking. Serve the casserole with the baked potato.

SPINACH MEALS

Spinach, as all Popeye fans know, is a good source of iron, but more important, it is a good source of dietary fibre and is very low in calories. A 4oz (115g) serving of cooked chopped spinach has only 35 calories and contains 7g dietary fibre.

It makes a good bed on which to serve other foods (for example, poached eggs) and so it can be turned into simple, quick meals. However, to add variety, one or two other methods of using spinach in meals have been included.

CHOPPED SPINACH – BASIC RECIPE

Calories 35; Fibre 7g

8oz (225g) fresh spinach, washed, *or* 4oz (115g) frozen chopped
   or cut-leaf spinach, thawed
salt and freshly ground pepper

If fresh spinach is used, cut out any coarse stalks, wash well and pack into a saucepan with only the water that clings to the leaves. Heat gently, turning the spinach occasionally, then bring to the boil and cook until soft, 10–15 minutes. Drain thoroughly and chop finely. Season to taste with salt and pepper.

If using thawed frozen spinach, do not add butter but heat very gently until simmering, adding 1 tablespoon water if necessary, and simmer for about 7 minutes, stirring frequently. Drain off any surplus liquid. Season to taste with salt and pepper. Use as a vegetable accompaniment or in one of the meals below.

SPINACH AND EGG BENEDICT WITH MUSHROOMS

Calories 150; Fibre 8g

1 portion chopped spinach (see above)
1 egg, size 3
2 tablespoons natural yogurt

1 teaspoon tomato purée
a dash of Worcestershire sauce
2oz (55g) button mushrooms
a sprig of parsley

Arrange the spinach on a hot serving plate. Poach the egg in water and place on top of the spinach. Mix the yogurt with the tomato purée and Worcestershire sauce and spoon over the egg. Poach the mushrooms in salted water or stock and serve with the spinach and egg, garnished with a sprig of parsley.

SPINACH WITH CREAMY HAM

Calories 175; Fibre 7g

2oz (55g) lean boiled ham
2 tablespoons low-fat natural yogurt
¼ teaspoon prepared mustard
1 portion chopped spinach (p. 114)

Trim off and discard any visible fat from the ham; chop the ham. Mix the yogurt with the mustard. Stir in the chopped ham. Arrange the hot spinach on a serving dish and spoon over the creamy ham topping. Serve at once.

SPINACH AND POACHED EGG ON TOAST

Calories 175; Fibre 9g

1oz (25g) slice wholemeal bread
1 portion chopped spinach (p. 114)
1 egg, size 3
paprika pepper
vinegar (optional)

Toast the bread on both sides. Pile the hot spinach on top of the toast. Poach the egg in water and place on the spinach. Garnish with a sprinkling of paprika pepper and serve with vinegar, if liked.

CHEESY SPINACH CRUMBLE

Calories 200; Fibre 8g

a pinch of grated nutmeg
1 portion chopped spinach (p. 114)
salt and pepper
4oz (115g) cottage cheese (natural or with onion and peppers)
½oz (15g) wholemeal breadcrumbs
1 tablespoon grated Parmesan cheese

Stir the grated nutmeg into the spinach, then arrange in a small oven-proof dish. Season the cottage cheese to taste and spoon over the spinach. Mix the breadcrumbs with the Parmesan cheese and sprinkle on top. Bake at 400°F, (200°C, gas 6) for 15 minutes or until the topping is crisp.

SPINACH OMELETTE WITH MUSHROOMS

Calories 225; Fibre 8g

2 eggs, size 3
1 portion chopped spinach (p. 114)
salt and pepper
¼oz (7g) low-fat spread
2oz (55g) button mushrooms

Separate the egg yolks from the whites. Mix the chopped spinach with the egg yolks, seasoning and 2 tablespoons water. Whisk the egg whites until stiff. Gently fold the egg whites into the spinach mixture. Grease a non-stick omelette pan with the low-fat spread and heat. Pour in the omelette mixture and cook over a moderate heat until the bottom is set. Place the pan under a grill to set and lightly brown the top of the omelette. Fold the omelette in half and turn out on to a warm serving dish. Poach the mushrooms in a little salted water or stock and serve with the omelette.

SPINACH WITH BEEFBURGERS AND TOMATO SAUCE

Calories 225; Fibre 8g

2 × 2oz (55g) frozen beefburgers
5oz (140g) canned tomatoes and juice
1 teaspoon dried onion flakes
salt and pepper
a dash of Worcestershire sauce
1 portion chopped spinach (p. 114)

Grill the beefburgers well on both sides so that much of the fat drips away. Mash the tomatoes with their juice and put in a small saucepan with the onion flakes, seasoning to taste and Worcestershire sauce. Bring to the boil and simmer gently for 5 minutes. Arrange the hot spinach on a serving plate. Place the beefburgers on top and pour the tomato sauce over them.

CHICKEN AND SPINACH WITH CARROTS

Calories 225; Fibre 10g

1 portion chopped spinach (p. 114)
4 tablespoons low-fat natural yogurt
1 teaspoon Worcestershire sauce
3oz (85g) cooked chicken
salt and pepper
paprika pepper
4oz (115g) carrots, sliced

Arrange the spinach in an ovenproof dish. Mix the yogurt with the Worcestershire sauce. Remove and discard any skin on the chicken, then cut into bite-size pieces. Mix the chicken with the yogurt and season to taste. Spoon the chicken mixture over the spinach, and heat through under a hot grill. Sprinkle over a little paprika. Boil the carrots and serve with the chicken and spinach dish.

FISH FLORENTINE LAYER

Calories 275; Fibre 10g

6oz (170g) haddock fillet or any white fish fillet, skinned
1 teaspoon lemon juice
salt and freshly ground pepper
1 portion chopped spinach (p. 114)
1oz (25g) fresh wholemeal breadcrumbs
½oz (15g) Cheddar cheese, finely grated
1 tablespoon chopped fresh parsley

Place the fish fillet in the bottom of a 1–1½ pint (600–900ml) oven-proof dish. Pour lemon juice over fish and season. Cover fish with the spinach. Mix together the breadcrumbs, cheese, parsley and salt and pepper to taste. Spoon the mixture on top of the spinach. Bake at 400°F (200°C, gas 6) for 20–30 minutes until breadcrumb topping is golden brown. Serve hot.

SPINACH WITH MINCED BEEF TOPPING

Calories 300; Fibre 11g

4oz (115g) raw minced beef
1 fresh tomato *or* 2oz (55g) canned tomatoes
1oz (25g) chopped onion
1oz (25g) mushrooms, chopped
½oz (15g) brown rice
4 tablespoons beef stock or water
salt and pepper
¼ level teaspoon dried mixed herbs
1 portion chopped spinach (p. 114)
2oz (55g) carrots, sliced

Fry the minced beef, without added fat, until well browned. Drain off and discard any fat which has been cooked out of the meat. Chop the fresh or canned tomato and add, with the chopped onion and mush-rooms, rice and stock or water to the meat in the pan. Season to taste with salt and pepper and add the herbs. Stir well and heat to simmering point. Cover and simmer gently for 30 minutes. Meanwhile, boil the carrots in lightly salted water until tender; then drain. Arrange the hot spinach on a serving plate and spoon the minced beef mixture on top. Serve with the boiled carrots.

WHOLE-WHEAT PASTA MEALS

Whole-wheat pasta includes spaghetti, spaghetti rings, marcaroni and lasagne, which gives plenty of scope for interesting meals as can be seen in this section. A 2oz (50g) dry-weight portion of any whole-wheat pasta, which when cooked gives a generous slimmer's portion, provides 5·7g fibre at a cost of 195 calories.

The fibre and calorie values of the pasta have been included in the total value for each meal in this section. However, should you want to add boiled whole-wheat pasta to any other meals, then use the figures above.

ITALIAN VEGETABLE SOUP

Calories 200; Fibre 8g

1 small onion (about 1oz, 25g), coarsely grated
1 carrot (about 2oz, 55g), coarsely grated
2oz (55g) parsnip, coarsely grated
½ chicken stock cube dissolved in ¼ pint (1·5dl) boiling water
¼ pint (1·5dl) tomato juice
1oz (25g) whole-wheat macaroni
2oz (55g) cabbage, finely shredded
salt and pepper
1 teaspoon chopped fresh parsley

Put the onion, carrot, parsnip, chicken stock, tomato juice and macaroni into a saucepan. Bring to the boil, cover and simmer gently for 15 minutes. Add the cabbage, bring back to the boil and cook, gently covered, for a further 5–10 minutes. Season to taste with salt and pepper and serve topped with the chopped parsley.

PASTA AND PRAWN SALAD

Calories 300; Fibre 7g

2oz (55g) whole-wheat macaroni or spaghetti rings
2oz (55g) peeled prawns
2oz (55g) button mushrooms, sliced

1 tablespoon low-calorie salad dressing
1 tablespoon low-fat natural yogurt
1 teaspoon lemon juice
salt and pepper
a few lettuce leaves
1 teaspoon chopped fresh parsley

Cook the macaroni or spaghetti rings in boiling salted water until just tender. Drain, rinse in cold water and drain again. Mix with the prawns and mushrooms. Blend together the salad dressing, yogurt and lemon juice. Add to the pasta mixture and stir until all the ingredients are thoroughly mixed. Season to taste. Arrange a bed of lettuce on a plate, spoon the salad on top and garnish with the chopped parsley.

PASTA WITH TUNA AND TOMATO SAUCE

Calories 325; Fibre 7g

2oz (55g) whole-wheat spaghetti or macaroni
5oz (140g) canned tomatoes
a pinch of dried basil or oregano
3½oz (100g) can tuna in brine, drained
a pinch of garlic salt
freshly ground pepper

Boil the pasta in salted water for about 12 minutes or until just tender. Meanwhile, purée the canned tomatoes in an electric blender or mash well with a fork. Place in a saucepan with the herbs. Flake the tuna and add to the tomato purée. Bring to the boil, reduce the heat and simmer for about 5 minutes. Add the garlic salt and pepper to taste. Drain the pasta. Serve the tuna and tomato sauce on the pasta.

MACARONI SCRAMBLE

Calories 350; Fibre 9g

2oz (55g) whole-wheat macaroni
2oz (55g) canned sweetcorn kernels mixed with red and green pepper
1 large egg (size 2)
2 tablespoons skimmed milk
salt and pepper

Boil the macaroni in salted water until tender, about 12 minutes. Drain and place in a non-stick saucepan with the sweetcorn. Beat the egg with the milk and seasoning to taste. Add to the saucepan. Heat gently, stirring continuously until the egg begins to set and becomes creamy. Turn out on to a serving dish and serve at once.

SPAGHETTI WITH CHILLI LENTIL SAUCE

Calories 375; Fibre 11g

1 teaspoon oil
1 small onion, peeled and chopped
$\frac{1}{2}$–1 teaspoon chilli powder
8oz (225g) canned tomatoes and juice
1oz (25g) lentils
1 level tablespoon tomato purée
salt and pepper
2oz (55g) whole-wheat spaghetti
1 level teaspoon chopped fresh parsley

Heat the oil in a small saucepan. Add the onion and fry gently until softened. Stir in the chilli powder. Chop the tomatoes and add to the pan with their juice; add the lentils, tomato purée and 2fl oz (55ml) water. Bring to the boil, reduce the heat, cover and simmer gently for about 30 minutes until the lentils have softened. Stir frequently and add more water if the mixture becomes too thick. Season to taste with salt and pepper. Boil the spaghetti in salted water until just tender, about 12 minutes. Drain the spaghetti and pile in the centre of a plate. Spoon the chilli lentil sauce around the spaghetti and sprinkle with chopped parsley.

PASTA WITH CHICKEN LIVER SAUCE

Calories 400; Fibre 8g

2oz (55g) whole-wheat spaghetti, macaroni or spaghetti rings
4oz (115g) chicken livers
¼ pint (1·5dl) chicken stock
2oz (55g) mushrooms, sliced
1 tablespoon dry sherry, optional
1 teaspoon tomato purée
salt and pepper
2 teaspoons wholemeal flour

Boil the pasta in salted water until just tender. Meanwhile, chop the chicken livers and place in a saucepan with the stock, mushrooms, sherry (if used), tomato purée and seasoning to taste. Bring to the boil, cover and simmer for 10 minutes. Blend the wholemeal flour with a little water and stir into the chicken liver sauce. Continue to heat, stirring continuously until the sauce is thickened. Drain the pasta and arrange in a circle on a plate. Spoon the sauce into the centre.

SPAGHETTI WITH FISH SAUCE

Calories 400; Fibre 8g

2oz (55g) whole-wheat spaghetti
6oz (170g) packet frozen cod in mushroom sauce
1oz (25g) frozen peas, cooked

Boil the spaghetti in salted water for about 12 minutes or until just tender. Heat the cod in mushroom sauce as directed. Boil the peas. Drain the spaghetti and arrange on a serving plate. Flake the fish into the mushroom sauce and stir in the peas. Spoon on top of the spaghetti and serve.

SPAGHETTI BOLOGNESE

Calories 400; Fibre 9g

2oz (55g) whole-wheat spaghetti

Sauce
4oz (115g) lean minced beef
1 small onion, peeled and finely chopped
1 stick celery, finely chopped
$\frac{1}{4}$ beef stock cube dissolved in $2\frac{1}{2}$fl oz (70ml) boiling water
salt and freshly ground pepper
a pinch of mixed herbs
1 teaspoon tomato purée
1oz (25g) frozen peas

Fry the minced beef in a non-stick saucepan until well browned. Drain off all the fat which has cooked out of the meat. Add the onion, celery and stock to the meat in the pan and bring to the boil, stirring. Reduce the heat, season to taste with salt and pepper and add the herbs and tomato purée. Cover and simmer gently for 40 minutes, stirring occasionally and adding more water if it begins to boil dry. Boil the spaghetti in salted water for about 12 minutes or until just tender. Drain and arrange around the edge of a serving dish. Stir the peas into the sauce and heat through for 5 minutes, then pour into the centre of the pasta.

KIDNEY LASAGNE

Calories 425; Fibre 13g

2oz (55g) whole-wheat lasagne
2 lamb's kidneys
1 small onion, peeled and sliced
2oz (55g) mushrooms, sliced
$\frac{1}{3}$ beef stock cube
1 teaspoon tomato purée
1 tablespoon wholemeal flour
salt and pepper

2oz (55g) frozen peas
4 tablespoons low-fat natural yogurt
a squeeze of lemon juice

Boil the lasagne in salted water for 15–17 minutes, stirring occasionally. Drain and rinse under running water. Skin, halve and remove cores from the kidneys. Chop and place in a pan with the onion, mushrooms, stock cube, tomato purée and ¼ pint (1·5dl) boiling water. Bring to the boil, cover and simmer for 15 minutes. Blend the flour with a little cold water and stir into the kidney sauce. Bring to the boil, stirring. Season with salt and pepper to taste and stir in the peas. Place half the lasagne in the base of a lightly greased ovenproof dish. Spoon over the kidney sauce and top with the remaining lasagne. Mix the yogurt with the lemon juice and season to taste. Spread over the lasagne. Cook in the oven at 400°F (200°C, gas 6) for 15 minutes or until heated through. Serve hot.

CHEESY-TOPPED VEGETABLE AND PASTA PIE

Calories 425; Fibre 17g

2oz (55g) whole-wheat spaghetti rings
2oz (55g) peas
2oz (55g) sweetcorn kernels
1 canned red pepper, sliced
5oz (142g) can condensed Golden Vegetable Soup
a dash of Worcestershire sauce
½oz (15g) wholemeal breadcrumbs
1 tablespoon grated Parmesan cheese

Boil the spaghetti rings in salted water until just tender. Drain and mix with the peas, sweetcorn and pepper. Blend the condensed soup with 3fl oz (85ml) water and stir into the pasta and vegetables with the Worcestershire sauce. Turn into a baking dish. Mix the breadcrumbs and cheese together and spoon over the top. Cook in the oven at 400°F (200°C, gas 6) for 20 minutes or until heated through.

MACARONI CHEESE WITH VEGETABLES

Calories 475; Fibre 12g

2oz (55g) whole-wheat macaroni
4oz (115g) frozen mixed vegetables
½oz (15g) wholemeal flour
¼ pint (1·5dl) skimmed milk
¼oz (7g) low-fat spread
salt and pepper
¼ teaspoon made mustard
1oz (25g) Edam cheese, grated

Boil the macaroni in salted water for 12 minutes or until tender; drain.
Cook the vegetables as directed and drain. Put the flour, milk and low-fat spread into a saucepan and heat, whisking continuously until it boils and thickens. Season to taste with salt and pepper. Add the mustard and half the cheese. Stir the macaroni and vegetables into the sauce. Turn into an ovenproof dish. Sprinkle over the remaining cheese. Cook in the oven at 400°F (200°C, gas 6) for 20 minutes or until the cheese is melted and bubbling.

BEAN LASAGNE

Calories 475; Fibre 22g

2oz (55g) whole-wheat lasagne
1 teaspoon low-fat spread
1 small onion, peeled and chopped
8oz (225g) baked beans with tomato sauce
a dash of Worcestershire sauce
2oz (55g) cottage cheese
2 tablespoons low-fat natural yogurt
salt and pepper
1 tablespoon grated Parmesan cheese

Boil the lasagne in salted water for 15 minutes. Drain and rinse under the cold water tap. Heat the low-fat spread in a non-stick pan and fry the onion over gentle heat until soft. Add the baked beans and Worcestershire sauce and heat through. Place half the lasagne in the bottom of a lightly greased ovenproof dish. Spoon in the hot baked bean mixture and top with the remaining lasagne. Mix the cottage cheese and yogurt together and season to taste. Spread over the lasagne to cover. Sprinkle on the grated Parmesan cheese. Place under a hot grill for 5–10 minutes until the Parmesan cheese is browned or cook at 400°F (200°C, gas 6) until the top is browned.

PEASE PUDDING MEALS

Peas are an excellent source of dietary fibre, so it is time to revive that good old favourite, pease pudding.

The basic recipe here gives quantities for one serving, but if you like pease pudding it would be sensible to multiply the ingredients and make at least four portions. Divide this into individual amounts, put each in a freezer carton or bag, freeze and use as required for the selection of meals listed below. To use, remove from carton or bag and place, still frozen, in a small ovenproof container. Cover and heat through in a moderate oven (375°F, 190°C, gas 5) for 30 minutes.

PEASE PUDDING – BASIC RECIPE

Calories 200; Fibre 7g

2oz (55g) dried split peas
1oz (25g) chopped onion
1 bay leaf, optional
salt
½ beef or ham stock cube
freshly ground black pepper

Cover the peas with boiling water and soak overnight. Drain, then put into a pan with the onion and bay leaf. Cover with fresh water, add a pinch of salt and the stock cube. Bring to the boil, then cover and simmer slowly until tender, about 1–1½ hours. Remove the bay leaf. Drain the peas and either sieve or purée in an electric blender or food processor. Stir in freshly ground pepper and salt to taste. Use in the meals set out below.

PEASE PUDDING SOUFFLÉ WITH TOMATO, ONION AND WATERCRESS SALAD

Calories 300; Fibre 9g

1 portion pease pudding (see above)
1 egg, size 3

salt and pepper
¼ teaspoon made mustard
1 tomato, sliced
1oz (25g) onion, sliced into rings
a small bunch of watercress

Place the pease pudding in a basin. Separate the egg yolk from the egg white and beat the yolk with seasoning to taste and the mustard into the pease pudding. Whisk the egg white until stiff, and gently fold in. Spoon the mixture into a 1½ pint (2l) ovenproof dish or soufflé dish and bake at 400°F (200°C, gas 6) for 20 minutes. Serve hot with a salad made from the sliced tomato, onion rings and sprigs of watercress.

BACON STEAK WITH PEASE PUDDING

Calories 325; Fibre 8g

3½oz (100g) bacon steak
1 small tomato
1 portion pease pudding (p. 128)

Grill the bacon steak well on both sides without added fat. Halve the tomato and warm through under the grill. Serve the well-grilled bacon steak with the tomato and pease pudding.

PEASE PUDDING WITH LAMB'S LIVER

Calories 450; Fibre 10g

4oz (115g) lamb's liver, sliced thinly
1 tablespoon bran
salt and freshly ground pepper
16 squirts low-calorie cooking spray (Limmit's Spray & Fry)
2oz (55g) Brussels sprouts
1 portion pease pudding (p. 128)

Wash the liver, coat with the bran, season with salt and pepper, and spray one side with 8 squirts of the cooking spray. Cook under a hot grill for 3 minutes, turn, spray the second side and cook for a further 3 minutes, or until just cooked through. Boil the Brussels sprouts. Serve the grilled liver with the pease pudding and sprouts.

PEASE PUDDING WITH COTTAGE CHEESE AND TOMATO TOPPING

Calories 325; Fibre 9g

1 portion pease pudding (p. 128)
4oz (115g) cottage cheese (natural or with chives)
2oz (55g) chopped fresh green pepper
salt and freshly ground pepper
1 tomato, sliced
1 tablespoon chopped fresh parsley

Spoon the pease pudding into a $1\frac{1}{2}$ pint (2l) ovenproof dish. Mix the cottage cheese with the chopped pepper and season to taste. Pile the cottage cheese mixture on to the pease pudding. Arrange the tomato slices over the cheese and season lightly. Bake at 400°F (200°C, gas 6) for 15–20 minutes or heat through under the grill. Serve hot, sprinkled with chopped parsley.

BAKED BEAN MEALS

In this section you will find many of the simplest no-nonsense sort of meals on the diet menus – and also many of those highest in dietary fibre content. Good old baked beans, canned in tomato sauce, are a splendid source of fibre at very moderate calorie cost. An 8oz (227g) can gives a generous serving for one, at a cost of only 160 calories.

Each meal gives quantities for one serving. At the end of this section, however, we have given recipes for a couple of baked bean meals which involve rather more ingredients and a little more time than you would want to spend on one meal. These are given in portions for four servings.

POACHED EGG WITH BAKED BEANS

Calories 250; Fibre 16g

1 large egg, size 2
8oz (225g) baked beans with tomato sauce

Poach the egg in water and serve on top of the heated baked beans.

BAKED BEANS ON TOAST

Calories 250; Fibre 19g

1 slice wholemeal bread (1¼oz, 35g)
1 teaspoon tomato purée
8oz (225g) baked beans with tomato sauce

Toast the bread and spread with the tomato purée. Spoon the heated beans over the toast.

BACON AND BAKED BEANS

Calories 275; Fibre 16g

2 rashers streaky bacon (¾oz, 20g each)
8oz (225g) baked beans with tomato sauce

Grill the bacon until crisp. Serve with the heated beans.

FISH FINGERS AND BAKED BEANS

Calories 275; Fibre 18g

2 cod fish fingers
1 large or 2 small tomatoes, halved
8oz (225g) baked beans with tomato sauce

Grill the fish fingers and tomatoes without added fat until the fish fingers are crisp on the outside and cooked through. Serve with the heated beans.

BAKED BEAN NEST

Calories 300; Fibre 13g

1 beefburger (2oz, 55g)
4oz (115g) baked beans with tomato sauce
1oz (25g) instant mashed potato, made up with boiling water as directed on packet

Grill the beefburger well and heat the beans. Pipe or spoon a ring of potato around the top edge of the cooked beefburger. Spoon the heated beans into the centre.

BAKED BEANS WITH CHEESE

Calories 300; Fibre 16g

6oz (170g) baked beans with tomato sauce
1oz (25g) Edam cheese, grated
1 canned red pepper, drained and chopped
½ teaspoon Worcestershire sauce
1 slice wholemeal bread (1¼oz, 35g), toasted

Heat the beans with the cheese, pepper and Worcestershire sauce over a gentle heat until hot and the cheese is melted. Serve the bean mixture on the hot toast.

BAKED BEANS AU GRATIN

Calories 300; Fibre 20g

2 tomatoes (2oz, 50g each)
8oz (225g) baked beans with tomato sauce
1oz (25g) wholemeal breadcrumbs
½oz (15g) Edam cheese, grated

Slice the tomatoes and place in a small gratin dish. Spoon over the heated beans. Mix the breadcrumbs with the cheese and sprinkle over beans. Grill until crisp and bubbly.

CHICKEN DRUMSTICKS WITH CURRIED BEANS

Calories 325; Fibre 16g

2 chicken drumsticks (3½oz, 100g each raw weight)
8oz (225g) baked beans with tomato sauce
1 teaspoon concentrated curry paste or curry powder

Grill the chicken drumsticks until cooked through. Heat the baked beans with the curry paste or powder. Remove and discard the skin from the chicken drumsticks and serve them with the curried beans.

WAGONS ROLL

Calories 325; Fibre 17g

1 wholemeal bread roll (2oz, 55g)
½oz (15g) low-fat spread
6oz (170g) baked beans with tomato sauce
salt and pepper
2 teaspoons sweet pickle
1 teaspoon slimmers' mayonnaise

Split the bread roll and spread with the low-fat spread. Mash the beans with seasoning to taste. Spread over the roll and top with the pickle and mayonnaise.

BAKED BEANS WITH MUSHROOMS

Calories 325; Fibre 23g

½oz (15g) low-fat spread
1 medium onion, peeled and chopped
4oz (115g) button mushrooms, trimmed
8oz (225g) baked beans with tomato sauce
1 teaspoon soy sauce
salt and pepper
1 slice wholemeal bread (1¼oz, 35g), toasted and cut in fingers

Melt the low-fat spread in a non-stick pan on a low heat. Add the onion and mushrooms and cook until soft. Add the beans, soy sauce and seasoning to taste. Serve with fingers of wholemeal toast.

CURRIED BEANS IN PITTA POCKET

Calories 325; Fibre 18g

8oz (225g) baked beans with tomato sauce
½oz (15g) sultanas
1 teaspoon curry powder
1 pitta bread (1⅝oz, 45g)

Heat the beans with the sultanas and curry powder until hot and bubbly. Halve the pitta bread and carefully cut again to make a pocket in each half. Fill the pockets with the bean mixture.

CHILLI BEEF AND BEANS

Calories 350; Fibre 13g

½ green pepper, seeds removed and chopped
3oz (85g) lean minced beef
1 small onion, peeled and chopped
4oz (115g) canned tomatoes
1 tablespoon tomato purée
½ teaspoon salt
1 teaspoon chilli powder
1 bay leaf
4oz (115g) baked beans with tomato sauce
2 crispbreads

Brown the green pepper, beef and onion in a non-stick saucepan. Drain off any fat which has cooked out of the meat. Add the tomatoes, tomato purée, salt, chilli powder and bay leaf. Cover and simmer for 40 minutes over a low heat. Add the beans and cook for a further 5 minutes. Serve with the crispbreads.

FRANKFURTER BEAN BAKE

Calories 350; Fibre 16g

8oz (225g) baked beans with tomato sauce
1 teaspoon tomato ketchup
½ teaspoon made mustard
1 teaspoon dried onion flakes
2oz (55g) frankfurters, sliced

Mix all the ingredients together, add 2 tablespoons water and spoon into a small ovenproof casserole. Cook, uncovered, in the oven at 350°F (180°C, gas 4) for 30 minutes.

CORNED BEEF WITH BAKED BEANS

Calories 350; Fibre 17g

3oz (85g) corned beef, sliced
8oz (225g) baked beans with tomato sauce
a few sprigs of watercress

Serve the corned beef with the heated baked beans. Garnish with the watercress.

QUICK AND EASY CASSOULET

Calories 375; Fibre 12g

1 rasher streaky bacon, rinds removed and diced
2oz (55g) garlic sausage, cubed
4oz (115g) canned tomatoes
4oz (115g) baked beans with tomato sauce
salt and pepper
$\frac{1}{4}$ teaspoon mixed dried herbs
1oz (25g) fresh wholemeal breadcrumbs

Place the bacon and garlic sausage in a non-stick saucepan and cook over a low heat until the fat runs and the bacon turns a crisp brown. Drain off any surplus fat. Add the tomatoes, beans and seasoning to taste. Transfer to a heatproof dish. Mix the herbs with the bread-crumbs and sprinkle over the bean mixture. Brown under a low grill for 5–10 minutes until crisp and bubbly.

OMELETTE AND BAKED BEANS

Calories 375; Fibre 16g

$\frac{1}{2}$oz (15g) low-fat spread
2 eggs, size 3, beaten
salt and pepper
8oz (225g) baked beans with tomato sauce

Melt the spread in a non-stick frying pan. Add the seasoned eggs and cook over a high heat until set. Fold the omelette in half and serve with the heated beans.

BEANS, SAUSAGE AND MASH

Calories 375; Fibre 21g

2 pork chipolata sausages
8oz (225g) baked beans with tomato sauce
1oz (25g) instant mashed potato made up with boiling water as directed
on the packet

Grill the sausages very thoroughly so that the maximum amount of fat runs off. Serve with the heated beans and mashed potato.

BEAN BURGER

Calories 400; Fibre 20g

1 beefburger (2oz, 55g)
1 wholemeal bread roll (2oz, 55g)
8oz (225g) baked beans with tomato sauce

Grill the beefburger thoroughly and toast the split bread roll. Place the burger on top of the bun and spoon over the heated beans.

SHEPHERDS' BEAN PIE

Calories 400; Fibre 21g

2oz (55g) lean minced beef
1 small onion (2oz, 55g), peeled and chopped
salt and pepper
8oz (225g) baked beans with tomato sauce
1oz (25g) instant mashed potato made up with boiling water as directed
on the packet

Cook the beef and onion with seasoning to taste in a non-stick pan until cooked and browned. Drain off any fat which has cooked out of the meat. Add the beans and heat through. Spoon into a small dish. Top with the mashed potato and grill until golden.

EASY BEAN GRILL

Calories 450; Fibre 17g

salt and pepper
1 lamb chump chop (5oz, 150g raw weight)
2 tomatoes, halved
8oz (225g) baked beans with tomato sauce

Season the chop and tomatoes and grill until the chop is cooked very thoroughly. Serve with the heated beans.

LIVER, BACON AND BEANS

Calories 500; Fibre 16g

4oz (115g) lamb's liver, sliced
1 teaspoon oil
2 rashers streaky bacon (¾oz, 20g each raw weight)
8oz (225g) baked beans with tomato sauce

Brush the liver with oil. Grill liver and bacon until the bacon is crisp. Serve with the heated beans.

HEARTY SAUSAGE AND BEAN SOUP
FOUR SERVINGS

Four portions: 900 calories; 40g fibre
Individual portion: 225 calories; 10g fibre

2 medium onions, peeled and chopped
6oz (170g) carrots, peeled and chopped
8oz (225g) canned tomatoes
2 chicken stock cubes

16oz (450g) baked beans with tomato sauce
4oz (115g) frankfurters, sliced
salt and pepper
4 tablespoons cornflour

Place the onions, carrots, tomatoes and stock cubes in a saucepan with
2¼ pints (1·25l) water and bring to the boil. Cover and simmer for 45
minutes. Add the baked beans, frankfurters and seasoning to taste.
Simmer for a further 10 minutes. Blend the cornflour with a little
water to make a smooth paste and blend into the hot soup. Cook for a
further 2–3 minutes, stirring constantly. Serve hot.

SAUCY BEAN RAREBIT – FOUR SERVINGS

Four portions: 1,100 calories; 80g fibre
Individual portion: 275 calories; 20g fibre

½oz (15g) low-fat spread
1 medium onion, peeled and chopped
1 garlic clove, crushed
1 green pepper, seeded and sliced
14oz (397g) can kidney beans, drained
16oz (450g) baked beans with tomato sauce
4 tablespoons tomato ketchup
1 tablespoon Worcestershire sauce
salt and pepper
4 slices (each 1¼oz, 35g) wholemeal bread, toasted

Melt the low-fat spread in a non-stick frying pan. Add the onion,
garlic and green pepper, and cook for 5 minutes until the onion is soft.
Stir in the kidney beans, baked beans, tomato ketchup, Worcestershire
sauce and seasoning to taste. Cook for a further 5 minutes, stirring
occasionally. Serve the bean rarebit on the slices of hot toast.

KIDNEY BEAN MEALS

The recipes in this section use fibre-rich kidney beans. These are mainly four-portion recipes so that you can store away the three remaining portions in freezer bags ready for future dieting meals.

To allow you a choice, here are the calorie and fibre contents of a variety of foods which you might serve with the kidney bean dishes. Add the figures of the food you choose as an accompaniment to that of the dish.

	Calories	Fibre (g)
Brown rice (2oz, 55g dry weight)	190	2
Energen Brancrisp crispbreads (2)	50	3
Lightly boiled cabbage (4oz, 115g)	20	3
Baked potato (6oz, 170g)	175	5

TUNA, TOMATO AND RED KIDNEY BEAN SAVOURY – TWO SERVINGS

Two portions: 400 calories; 16g fibre
Individual portion: 200 calories; 8g fibre

8oz (227g) can peeled tomatoes
1 tablespoon (15ml) tomato purée
7·9oz (223g) can Batchelor's Red Kidney Beans
freshly ground pepper
$\frac{1}{4}$ level teaspoon curry powder
7oz (198g) can Sainsbury's Tuna in Brine
4oz (115g) frozen whole green beans, per serving

Put the contents of the can of tomatoes into a pan and break down with a fork. Add the tomato purée, drained kidney beans, ground pepper and curry powder and heat through. Drain and flake the tuna, add to the tomatoes and beans and heat through. Cook the frozen green beans. Serve the tuna, tomato and red kidney bean savoury with the green beans.

PORK AND BEAN CASSEROLE – FOUR SERVINGS

Four portions: 900 calories; 30g fibre
Individual portion: 225 calories; 8g fibre

12oz (340g) pork fillet
1 large onion, peeled and chopped
1 canned red pepper, sliced
3oz (85g) dried red kidney beans, soaked overnight
1oz (25g) haricot beans, soaked overnight
7oz (200g) canned tomatoes
salt and pepper
$\frac{1}{2}$ pint (3dl) stock
$\frac{1}{4}$ pint (1·5dl) cider

Cut the pork into small pieces. Put all ingredients into a large saucepan, bring to the boil. Boil for 10 minutes, then cover and simmer gently for 1–1$\frac{1}{2}$ hours until cooked. Remove the lid for the last 15 minutes to reduce the sauce.

BEAN AND BEEF STEW – FOUR SERVINGS

Four portions: 1,000 calories; 24g fibre
Individual portion: 250 calories; 11g fibre

1 tablespoon oil
12oz (340g) very lean stewing beef, diced
1 large onion, peeled and sliced
1 tablespoon flour
$\frac{1}{2}$ pint (3dl) brown stock
2 teaspoons tomato purée
salt and pepper
a pinch of mixed herbs
15oz (425g) can red kidney beans, drained

Put the oil, beef and onion into a large saucepan and heat until slightly browned. Sprinkle on the flour and stir in the stock. Bring to the boil, add the remaining ingredients, cover and simmer for about 1$\frac{1}{2}$–2 hours until the beef is cooked.

KIDNEY BEAN SALAD – FOUR SERVINGS

Four portions: 1,000 calories; 42g fibre
Individual portion: 250 calories; 11g fibre

4oz (115g) dried red kidney beans, soaked overnight *or* 15oz (425g)
  can red kidney beans, drained
4oz (115g) frozen French beans
1 cauliflower (about 1lb, 450g)
1 small onion, peeled and finely chopped
4oz (115g) Edam cheese, cubed
juice of 1 lemon
2 tablespoons olive oil
3 tablespoons Waistline Oil-Free French Dressing
salt and pepper

Drain the soaked kidney beans, place in a saucepan and cover with fresh water. Bring to the boil, add a little salt, cover and simmer for about 1 hour until tender. Drain and rinse with cold water. If using canned beans, drain and rinse. Cook the French beans in boiling salted water for 2 minutes, then drain. Break the cauliflower into florets. Mix the kidney beans, French beans, cauliflower florets, onion and cheese together in a salad bowl. Mix the lemon juice, olive oil and French dressing together. Pour over the salad and toss well. Leave to stand for 30 minutes, then toss again and check seasoning before serving.

CHILLI CON CARNE – FOUR SERVINGS

Four portions: 1,200 calories; 28g fibre
Individual portion: 300 calories; 7g fibre

1lb (450g) lean minced beef
28oz (795g) canned tomatoes
1 large onion, peeled and chopped
15oz (425g) can red kidney beans
salt and pepper
chilli powder to taste (about 2 teaspoons)

Brown the minced beef in a non-stick pan and drain off the fat. Heat the tomatoes in a large saucepan. Add the mince, onion, drained red kidney beans, and seasoning and chilli powder to taste. Bring to the boil, cover and simmer very gently for about 1 hour.

HI-FI OMELETTES

CORN OMELETTE

Calories 250; Fibre 6g

2 eggs, size 3
2 tablespoons milk
a dash of Worcestershire sauce
salt and pepper
2oz (55g) sweetcorn
1oz (25g) peas

Beat the eggs, milk, Worcestershire sauce and seasoning together. Pour into a non-stick omelette pan and cook gently until almost set. Add the sweetcorn and peas and heat under the grill for a few minutes. Fold the omelette and serve.

VEGETABLE OMELETTE

Calories 400; Fibre 12g

½oz (15g) butter
½ small onion, chopped
1oz (25g) green pepper, chopped
7½oz (213g) can red kidney beans, drained
2 eggs (size 3)
a pinch of dried mixed herbs
salt and pepper

Melt the butter in an omelette or frying pan and fry the onion and pepper until softened. Stir in the beans and heat through. Beat the eggs, herbs, seasoning and 2 tablespoons water together. Pour over the vegetables. Cook gently, forking up the cooked mixture frequently to let the raw egg mixture get to the bottom of the pan. When the egg is just set, fold in half and serve.

HI-FI SALADS

The average salad isn't necessarily as good a source of fibre (or anything else of much nutritional value) as people imagine. Professor Peter Van Soest – one of the top fibre experts in the USA – has commented that 'salad is little more than packaged water'.

Combine on your plate a generous quantity of lettuce and cucumber and radishes, a spring onion or two and some watercress and you are unlikely to be eating much more than one gram of dietary fibre.

The salads in this section are specially devised to make a realistic contribution to your daily fibre intake, and at modest calorie cost.

We haven't included the calorie cost of salad dressings, but we have indicated where they might be nice. Add the modest calorie cost to that of your hi-fi salad. Here is a list of commercial low-calorie salad dressings for you to choose from, followed by some recipes for home-made salad dressings.

Dietade Low-Calorie Salad Dressing without Oil	negligible calories per tablespoon
Waistline Oil-Free French Dressing	5 calories per tablespoon
Heinz Slimway Low Calorie Salad Dressing	20 calories per tablespoon
Waistline Vinegar and Oil Dressing	25 calories per tablespoon

HOME-MADE SALAD DRESSINGS

TANGY TOMATO DRESSING

Calories 5

1 tablespoon tomato juice
1 teaspoon Worcestershire sauce
1 teaspoon lemon juice or vinegar
salt and pepper

Blend all the dressing ingredients together.

YOGURT MINT DRESSING

Calories 10

1 tablespoon low-fat natural yogurt
1 teaspoon lemon juice
½ teaspoon chopped fresh mint or ¼ teaspoon concentrated
   mint sauce
salt and pepper

Blend all the dressing ingredients together.

TOMATO YOGURT SALAD DRESSING

Calories 15

1 tablespoon tomato juice
1 tablespoon low-fat natural yogurt
a pinch of sugar
a pinch of dry mustard
salt and pepper

Blend all the dressing ingredients together.

HI-FI SALADS

PRAWN AND PEPPER SALAD

Calories 100; Fibre 5g

4oz (115g) green pepper, cored, seeded and chopped
2oz (55g) beansprouts
4oz (115g) tomatoes, quartered
2oz (55g) prawns
1 tablespoon lemon juice

Combine all the ingredients and sprinkle with the lemon juice.
   Suggested dressing: tomato yogurt dressing (above).

BEETROOT AND MUSHROOM SALAD WITH EGG

Calories 125; Fibre 4g

3oz (85g) cooked beetroot, peeled and cubed
2oz (55g) mushrooms, thinly sliced
1 egg (size 3), hard-boiled, quartered lengthwise
sprigs of watercress for garnish

Mix beetroot and mushrooms together and serve with hard-boiled egg.
Garnish with sprigs of watercress.
    Suggested dressing: tangy tomato dressing (p. 145).

BEETROOT, CARROT AND SHRIMP SALAD

Calories 125; Fibre 8g

2oz (55g) cooked beetroot, peeled and finely diced
3oz (85g) carrot, peeled and finely diced
1 tablespoon low-fat natural yogurt
1 teaspoon horseradish relish
2oz (55g) watercress sprigs
2oz (55g) beansprouts
2oz (55g) canned shrimps, drained

Put the beetroot and carrot in a basin. Mix the yogurt with the horseradish relish and stir into the beetroot and carrot. Spoon it into the
centre of a shallow dish. Surround with watercress sprigs and
beansprouts. Add the shrimps or serve separately.

HAM WITH TOMATO AND FRENCH BEAN SALAD

Calories 150; Fibre 3g

2 tomatoes, sliced
2oz (55g) whole French beans, fresh or frozen, slightly undercooked

1 tablespoon chopped chives or spring onions
2oz (55g) lean ham

Arrange the tomatoes and beans on a plate, sprinkle with chives or spring onions. Trim off and discard any fat from the ham and serve with the salad.

Suggested dressing: Dietade Low-Calorie Salad Dressing without Oil *or* Waistline Oil-Free French Dressing *or* tangy tomato dressing (p. 145).

CAULIFLOWER, PEAS, PEPPER AND CHEESE SALAD

Calories 150; Fibre 4g

2oz (55g) cauliflower sprigs
2oz (55g) cooked peas, fresh or frozen
1oz (25g) chopped green pepper
1oz (25g) Edam cheese, cubed or grated
1 tablespoon Heinz Slimway Low Calorie Salad Dressing
salt and pepper

Mix all the ingredients together and season to taste with salt and pepper.

CHICKEN WITH CELERY, APPLE AND WATERCRESS SALAD

Calories 150; Fibre 4g

5oz (140g) apple, cored and thinly sliced
1 teaspoon lemon juice
2oz (55g) celery, thinly sliced
2oz (55g) watercress sprigs
2oz (55g) lean roast chicken, sliced

Toss the apple slices in the lemon juice and combine with the celery and watercress. Remove and discard any skin from the sliced chicken and serve with the salad.

Suggested dressing: 1 tablespoon Waistline Vinegar and Oil Dressing *or* Heinz Slimway Low-Calorie Salad Dressing.

COLESLAW WITH FISH

Calories 150; Fibre 5g

3oz (85g) firm white cabbage, shredded
2oz (55g) carrot, grated
1 stick celery, finely chopped
1 tablespoon chopped chives or spring onion
1 tablespoon low-calorie salad dressing
1 tablespoon low-fat natural yogurt
a pinch of curry powder
4oz (115g) poached white fish, cooled and flaked

Mix the cabbage, carrot, celery and chives together in a basin. Blend the low-calorie salad dressing with the yogurt and curry powder. Add to the vegetables and mix well. Lightly stir in the flaked fish and serve.

PEACH AND COTTAGE CHEESE SALAD

Calories 175; Fibre 4g

2oz (55g) Chinese cabbage leaves, thinly sliced crossways
2oz (55g) mushrooms, thinly sliced
4oz (115g) fresh peach, sliced
1 tablespoon Waistline Oil-Free French Dressing
1 tablespoon low-fat natural yogurt
4oz (115g) cottage cheese
1oz (25g) parsley, finely chopped

Combine the cabbage, mushrooms and peach. Add the oil-free dressing and yogurt and toss well together. Mix the cottage cheese with the parsley and serve with the salad vegetables.

HAM WITH COLESLAW

Calories 175; Fibre 6g

3oz (85g) firm white cabbage, shredded
1 tablespoon finely chopped onion
2oz (55g) carrot, grated
1 tablespoon Oil-Free French Dressing
2oz (55g) lean boiled ham, sliced
2 medium tomatoes, halved and sliced

Mix the cabbage with the onion, carrot and dressing. Serve with the ham and tomatoes.

FRUIT AND CABBAGE SALAD

Calories 175; Fibre 13g

1oz (25g) dried apricots, chopped
½oz (15g) raisins
2 tablespoons orange juice
4oz (115g) eating apple
1 tablespoon lemon juice
3oz (85g) white or red cabbage, chopped
1 stick celery, chopped

Soak the dried apricots and raisins in the orange juice for half an hour. Core and chop the apple and toss in the lemon juice until coated to prevent discoloration. Add the fruits to the chopped cabbage and celery and toss well to mix.

BEAN-STUFFED TOMATOES

Calories 175; Fibre 16g

2 large tomatoes, 4oz (115g) each
1 stick celery, finely chopped
6oz (170g) baked beans with tomato sauce

salt and pepper
2oz (55g) white cabbage, chopped

Cut a lid off both tomatoes and remove the centre pulp; chop finely.
Mix with the celery, beans and seasoning to taste. Pile back into the
tomato cases. Serve on a bed of chopped white cabbage.

POTATO, BEETROOT AND PRAWN SALAD

Calories 200; Fibre 5g

3oz (85g) cooked beetroot, peeled and diced
4oz (115g) new potatoes, boiled and diced
1 small onion, peeled and finely chopped
1oz (25g) parsley, finely chopped
1 tablespoon Waistline Oil-Free French Dressing
2oz (55g) prawns

Mix the beetroot and potatoes together. Add the onion, parsley and
dressing and toss together until well mixed. Top with the prawns.

ORANGE, BROAD BEAN, CELERY AND COTTAGE CHEESE SALAD

Calories 200; Fibre 7g

1 medium orange, peeled and sliced
2oz (55g) broad beans, boiled and drained
2oz (55g) celery, thinly sliced
½oz (15g) almonds, chopped
2oz (55g) cottage cheese

Combine the orange, broad beans and celery. Sprinkle with almonds
and serve with the cottage cheese.
    Suggested dressing: yogurt mint dressing (p. 146) *or* 1 tablespoon
Waistline Oil-Free French Dressing.

POTATO AND TUNA SALAD

Calories 200; Fibre 7g

4oz (115g) new potatoes, boiled and diced
1 tablespoon Waistline Oil-Free French Dressing
1 tablespoon low-fat natural yogurt
salt and pepper
2oz (55g) fresh or thawed frozen garden peas
1oz (25g) red pepper, chopped
1 tablespoon chopped chives
2oz (55g) tuna in brine, drained and flaked

Put the potatoes while still warm in a basin. Mix the oil-free dressing, yogurt and seasoning together and stir into the warm potatoes. Leave to get cold, then add the peas, red pepper, chives and tuna. Toss well and serve.

SUMMER SALAD

Calories 200; Fibre 8g

2oz (55g) new turnips, grated
2oz (55g) new carrots, grated
2oz (55g) cooked peas
1oz (25g) raisins
1 hard-boiled egg, thickly sliced

Mix the grated vegetables with peas and raisins and top with slices of egg.

Suggested dressing: 1 tablespoon Waistline Low-Calorie Vinegar and Oil Dressing *or* Heinz Slimway Low-Calorie Salad Dressing.

SPINACH, CARROT, NUT AND TURKEY SALAD

Calories 200; Fibre 11g

4oz (115g) spinach leaves, shredded
2oz (55g) carrots, coarsely grated

½oz (15g) almonds, chopped
2oz (55g) roast turkey

Mix the spinach leaves with carrots and almonds. Add dressing if wished and serve with turkey.

Suggested dressing: tangy tomato dressing (p. 145).

BROCCOLI, RED PEPPER AND GRAPE SALAD WITH CORNED BEEF

Calories 225; Fibre 5g

4oz (115g) broccoli, fresh or frozen, cooked and well drained
1 canned red pepper, drained and chopped
4oz (115g) white grapes
1 tablespoon Waistline Oil-Free French Dressing
2oz (55g) corned beef, sliced

Mix the broccoli and red pepper. Halve the grapes, remove seeds and add to the vegetables, with the dressing. Toss well and chill for 30 minutes. Serve with the corned beef.

SAVOY SALAD

Calories 225; Fibre 7g

4oz (115g) Savoy cabbage, thinly sliced
1oz (25g) currants
4oz (115g) fresh or canned pineapple in natural juice, cut into small chunks
1 tablespoon natural pineapple juice
2oz (55g) lean roast chicken

Combine Savoy cabbage, currants, pineapple and juice. Remove and discard any skin from the chicken. Cut the meat into bite-size pieces and mix with the remaining ingredients.

LEEK, KIDNEY BEAN AND CAULIFLOWER SALAD WITH SMOKED MACKEREL

Calories 225; Fibre 8g

4oz (115g) leeks (white part only), sliced
2oz (55g) canned red kidney beans, rinsed and well drained
2oz (55g) raw cauliflower sprigs
1 tablespoon lemon juice or wine vinegar
2oz (55g) smoked mackerel

Mix the leeks with the kidney beans and cauliflower sprigs. Sprinkle with lemon juice or vinegar, and toss well. Serve smoked mackerel separately.

AMERICAN BEAN SALAD AND COTTAGE CHEESE

Calories 225; Fibre 7g

half 1lb 1oz (482g) can Green Giant American Bean Salad
4oz (113g) carton Eden Vale Cottage Cheese with Onion and Peppers

Drain the bean salad and serve with the cottage cheese.

TWO-BEAN SALAD WITH COTTAGE CHEESE

Calories 250; Fibre 12g

2oz (55g) canned red kidney beans, rinsed and drained
2oz (55g) runner beans, cooked
2oz (55g) sweetcorn kernels
½oz (15g) peanuts
2 tablespoons Waistline Oil-Free French Dressing
2oz (55g) cottage cheese
1 tablespoon finely chopped parsley
1 teaspoon chopped chives *or* spring onion

Mix together the kidney beans, runner beans, sweetcorn and peanuts, and toss in the French dressing. Serve with cottage cheese mixed with the parsley and chives or spring onion.

NUTTY COLESLAW

Calories 275; Fibre 13g

4oz (115g) firm white cabbage, shredded
2oz (55g) carrot, grated
2oz (55g) fresh peas *or* frozen peas, cooked
2oz (55g) sweetcorn kernels, cooked
1oz (25g) walnut pieces, roughly chopped
yogurt mint dressing (p. 146)

Mix all the prepared vegetables and nuts together in a bowl. Stir in the yogurt mint dressing and serve.

BOLOGNA AND BEAN SALAD

Calories 300; Fibre 12g

one-third 10oz (283g) can Granose Bologna
1 tomato, sliced
one-third 1lb 1oz (482g) can Green Giant American Bean Salad
4 black or green olives
2 Ideal Bran Crispbreads

Slice the Bologna thinly and arrange in a circle around a serving plate. Pile the bean salad in the centre. Garnish with the sliced tomato and olives. Chill before serving. Accompany with the crispbreads.

KIDNEY BEAN, ONION, APPLE AND CHEESE SALAD

Calories 300; Fibre 10g

3oz (85g) canned red kidney beans, drained and rinsed
2 spring onions, chopped
4oz (115g) eating apple
1 tablespoon (15ml) lemon juice
1½oz (40g) mature Cheddar cheese, diced
2 tablespoons (30ml) oil-free French dressing

Mix the kidney beans and chopped spring onions together in a bowl. Core and chop the apple then toss in the lemon juice. Add the apple, diced cheese and oil-free French dressing to the kidney beans and onion and toss well. Chill before serving.

CORNED BEEF SALAD

Calories 350; Fibre 15g

half 1lb 1oz (482g) can Green Giant American Bean Salad
half 7oz (198g) can sweetcorn kernels
2oz (55g) corned beef, diced
2 tablespoons (30ml) oil-free French dressing
few lettuce leaves
1 Ideal Bran Crispbread

Drain the bean salad and the sweetcorn kernels and place in a bowl. Add the diced corned beef and the dressing and toss well together. Serve on a bed of lettuce. Serve the crispbread with the salad.

HI-FI SOUP SNACK MEALS

Some soups can provide super fibre-rich meals. Here we give basic recipes for pea, lentil and sweetcorn soups and show you how you can use them to make a whole variety of easy F-Plan meals.

No one wants to go to the bother of making their own soup for one meal, so we have given quantities for four portions with each basic recipe. The idea is that you should divide the quantity into four, use one and deep freeze the other three in individual rigid plastic containers – empty cartons, for instance.

In the meal section, beneath each soup, we show how adding a bit of this and that can ring the changes on your basic soup.

In giving the calorie and fibre count for each soup we have included one slice of wholemeal bread ($1\frac{1}{4}oz$, 35g) to eat with it. This is not buttered. If you spread your bread, add the following calories:

$\frac{1}{4}$oz (7g) butter or margarine	50 calories
$\frac{1}{4}$oz (7g) low-fat spread (Outline, St Ivel Gold)	25 calories
$\frac{1}{4}$oz (7g) peanut butter	45 calories
$\frac{1}{2}$oz (15g) cheese spread (a good alternative for dieters)	35 calories

LENTIL SOUP – BASIC RECIPE, FOUR PORTIONS

Four portions: 600 calories; 25g fibre
Individual portion: 150 calories; 6g fibre
Individual portion plus slice of wholemeal
   bread: 225 calories; 9g fibre

Basic four-portion recipe to make and freeze for lentil soup meals.

6oz (170g) dried lentils
2 pints (1l) water or stock
1 lemon, rind and juice
1 clove garlic, crushed
4oz (115g) onions, chopped
2oz (55g) carrot, chopped
1 clove
salt and freshly ground black pepper

Soak the lentils in water or stock overnight. Put the lemon rind and juice in a heavy-based saucepan and gently sweat the garlic, onions and carrot with the lid on for about 10 minutes, until softened. Add the lentils with the soaking liquid, clove and seasoning. Cover, bring to the boil. Boil for 10 minutes, then simmer for 1–2 hours until the lentils are soft and mushy. For a smooth soup, blend the soup in a liquidizer, first removing the clove.

LENTIL AND VEGETABLE SOUP

Calories 250; Fibre 12g

4oz (115g) tomatoes, chopped
2oz (55g) mushrooms, chopped
1 portion basic lentil soup (see previous page)

Simmer the vegetables in the soup for about 5 minutes. Eat with wholemeal bread.

CURRY-FLAVOURED LENTIL SOUP

Calories 250; Fibre 10g

1 portion basic lentil soup (see previous page)
2oz (55g) apple, chopped
½ teaspoon curry powder
2 teaspoons chutney

Simmer all the ingredients in the soup for about 5 minutes. Eat with wholemeal bread.

LENTIL, CHICKEN AND LEEK SOUP

Calories 275; Fibre 11g

1oz (25g) white chicken or turkey meat, cooked and chopped
2oz (55g) leeks, sliced
1 portion basic lentil soup (see previous page)

Simmer the poultry meat and leeks in the soup for about 5 minutes. Eat with wholemeal bread.

PEA SOUP – BASIC RECIPE, FOUR PORTIONS

Four portions: 520 calories; 32g fibre
Individual portion: 130 calories; 8g fibre
Individual portion plus slice of wholemeal
   bread: 205 calories; 11g fibre

Basic four-portion recipe to make and freeze for pea soup meals.

6oz (170g) dried peas
2 pints (1l) water or stock
4oz (115g) onion, chopped
2oz (55g) celery, chopped
$\frac{1}{4}$ teaspoon dried sage or savory
2 tablespoons fresh chopped parsley
salt and freshly ground black pepper

Soak the peas overnight in the water or stock. Put about two tablespoons of the soaking water in the base of a heavy saucepan and add the onion and celery; cover and gently sweat the vegetables for about 10 minutes. Do not allow to burn. Then pour in the rest of the liquid and peas. Add the herbs and seasoning. Bring to the boil and simmer, covered, for about 2 hours until the peas are soft. For a smooth creamy soup, blend in a liquidizer.

One slice of wholemeal bread (see introduction to the soup section) is included in both the calorie and fibre count of each of these snack meals.

CHUNKY PEA SOUP

Calories 250; Fibre 13g

1 portion basic pea soup (see above)
2oz (55g) carrots, chopped
2oz (55g) apple, chopped
1oz (25g) low-fat natural yogurt

Simmer the carrot and apple in the soup for about 5 minutes. Stir in the yogurt before serving. Eat with wholemeal bread.

PEA SOUP WITH HAM

Calories 275; Fibre 11g

1 portion basic pea soup (see previous page)
1oz (25g) lean boiled ham, chopped

Simmer the ham in the soup for about 5 minutes. Eat with wholemeal bread.

PEA SOUP WITH LEEK AND EGG

Calories 300; Fibre 14g

1 portion basic pea soup (see previous page)
3oz (85g) leeks, sliced thinly
1 egg (size 5 or 6)

Simmer the leeks in the soup for about 5 minutes. Hard-boil the egg, and chop. Crumble the chopped egg into the soup before serving. Eat with wholemeal bread.

SWEETCORN SOUP – BASIC RECIPE, FOUR PORTIONS

Four portions: 260 calories; 12g fibre
Individual portion: 65 calories; 3g fibre
Individual portion plus slice of wholemeal
** bread: 140 calories; 6g fibre**

Basic four-portion recipe to make and freeze for sweetcorn soup meals.

6oz (170g) sweetcorn kernels, frozen or canned
1½ pints (9dl) water or stock
4oz (115g) onion, chopped

½ teaspoon sugar
½ teaspoon dry mustard powder
1 tablespoon lemon juice
3 drops tabasco sauce
1 tablespoon Worcestershire sauce
salt and freshly ground black pepper
½ pint (3dl) skimmed milk, additional to daily allowance

Put all the ingredients, except the milk, into a saucepan. Bring to the boil, cover and simmer for about 30 minutes. Add the milk. If preferred, blend until smooth in a liquidizer – otherwise leave chunky.

One slice of wholemeal bread (see introduction to the soup section) is included in both the calorie and fibre count of each of these snack meals.

SWEETCORN SOUP WITH CHICKEN AND BEANSPROUTS

Calories 175; Fibre 7g

1oz (25g) cooked chicken or turkey meat, chopped
1 portion basic sweetcorn soup (see left)
1oz (25g) fresh beansprouts

Simmer the chicken or turkey in the soup for about 5 minutes, then stir in the beansprouts. Leave them crisp. Eat with wholemeal bread.

SWEETCORN SOUP WITH VEGETABLES

Calories 175; Fibre 7g

1 portion basic sweetcorn soup (see left)
2oz (55g) tomato, chopped
4oz (115g) courgettes, sliced

Add the vegetables to the soup and simmer for about 5 minutes. Eat with wholemeal bread.

SWEETCORN SOUP WITH CRAB

Calories 200; Fibre 6g

1oz (25g) canned crab meat
1oz (25g) apple, chopped
1 portion basic sweetcorn soup (p. 160)

Add the crab meat and apple to the soup and simmer for about 5 minutes. Eat with wholemeal bread.

SWEETCORN CHOWDER

Calories 200; Fibre 6g

2oz (55g) any white fish, cooked and flaked, *or* peeled prawns
1 portion basic sweetcorn soup (p. 160)

Add the flaked fish or prawns to the soup and simmer for about 5 minutes. Eat with wholemeal bread.

HI-FI CRISPBREADS

All these crispbread snacks are served on Energen Brancrisp crisp-breads. We have included two – supplying 50 calories and 2·6g fibre in total – in the calorie and fibre count for each meal. Don't use other crispbreads because the alternative well-known brands are lower in fibre content.

These snacks, perhaps eaten with fruit from the daily allowance, could be useful for those who like to follow a little-and-often pattern of eating. Alternatively they could provide a suppertime snack for those with calories to spare, or even a very light lunch for those who like to save most of their calories for the evening.

CURRIED CHEESE

Calories 125; Fibre 3g

4 tablespoons cottage cheese
2 teaspoons curry paste
2 teaspoons sweet pickle

Mix the cottage cheese and curry paste and spread over the crispbreads. Spoon the pickle in the centre of each.

CHEESE AND SWEETCORN PICKLE

Calories 125; Fibre 4g

½oz (15g) or 1 triangle cheese spread
1oz (25g) cucumber, sliced
1oz (25g) corn relish

Spread the crispbreads with the cheese spread. Top with the cucumber slices and the corn relish.

PEANUT BUTTER AND CRESS

Calories 150; Fibre 4g

4 teaspoons peanut butter
1 stick celery, chopped
½ carton mustard and cress

Mix the peanut butter and celery. Spread on the crispbreads and garnish with the mustard and cress.

CHEESE AND ONION

Calories 150; Fibre 4g

1 small onion, chopped
1oz (25g) cheese spread
8 potato crisps

Mix the onion and cheese spread and four of the crisps. Spread on the crispbreads and crush the other crisps. Sprinkle over the top.

PIQUANT FISH

Calories 150; Fibre 5g

3oz (85g) cod or haddock
1 tablespoon low-calorie tartare sauce (Waistline)
1 tablespoon peas, cooked
ground pepper
2 lemon wedges

Poach the fish, flake and cool. Mix it with the dressing, peas and pepper. Spread on the crispbreads and top with lemon wedges.

CHOCOLATE AND BANANA

Calories 150; Fibre 5g

2 teaspoons chocolate spread
1 small banana (4½oz, 130g)
1 teaspoon lemon juice

Spread a teaspoonful of chocolate spread on each crispbread. Slice the banana and arrange on top of the crispbreads. Sprinkle with the lemon juice.

PRAWN AND CELERY

Calories 150; Fibre 5g

2 sticks celery
1 tablespoon low-calorie salad dressing
2oz (55g) prawns

Finely chop the celery and mix with the salad dressing. Spread over the crispbreads and top with the prawns.

HAM AND PEA

Calories 150; Fibre 5g

1 large slice lean ham (1oz, 25g)
½ small onion, finely chopped
1oz (25g) peas, cooked
1 tablespoon low-calorie salad dressing

Chop the ham and mix it with the other ingredients. Spread on the crispbreads.

FRUIT, VEGETABLES AND CHEESE

Calories 150; Fibre 7g

1oz (25g) peas, cooked
1oz (25g) canned sweetcorn
1oz (25g) low-fat curd cheese
¼oz (7g) raisins

Mix all the ingredients together and spread on the crispbreads.

EGG AND SWEETCORN

Calories 175; Fibre 4g

1 hard-boiled egg (size 3)
1oz (25g) canned sweetcorn
1 tablespoon low-calorie salad dressing
salt and pepper

Chop the egg. Mix with the other ingredients and spread over the crispbreads.

CHICKEN AND MUSHROOM

Calories 175; Fibre 4g

2oz (55g) cooked chicken meat, chopped
4 button mushrooms, chopped
salt and pepper
1 tablespoon low-calorie salad dressing
1 tablespoon chopped walnuts

Mix the chicken, mushrooms, seasoning and salad dressing together. Spread on the crispbreads and garnish with the chopped nuts.

COTTAGE CHEESE, RAISIN AND APPLE

Calories 175; Fibre 5g

2oz (55g) cottage cheese
½oz (15g) raisins
4oz (115g) eating apple, cored and sliced

Mix the cottage cheese and raisins and spread over the crispbreads. Cover with the apple slices.

PORK AND APPLE

Calories 175; Fibre 7g

2oz (55g) cooked lean pork
4 prunes (soaked if dried)
½oz (15g) low-fat spread
1 tablespoon apple sauce

Chop the pork finely. Remove the stones from the prunes and chop the flesh. Add to the pork. Spread the low-fat spread on the crispbreads, and then the pork mixture. Top with a little apple sauce.

COTTAGE CHEESE WITH APRICOTS

Calories 225; Fibre 14g

4oz (113g) carton Eden Vale Cottage Cheese with Pineapple
2oz (56g) Whitworths No-need-to-soak Dried Apricots

Mix together the cottage cheese with the chopped dried apricots. Serve with the crispbreads.

MEALS ON TOAST

The meals in this section are all served on two slices of wholemeal or whole-wheat bread, toasted. Maximum total weight for the two slices must be 2½oz (70g). The calories for this quantity of bread, and the 6g fibre they supply, are included in the totals for each meal. If you use high bran bread, add another 2g fibre to the total for each meal.

With some meals we have relied on the bread alone to provide dietary fibre. With others we have added more dietary fibre in the ingredients used for the topping.

Some of these meals on toast are as simple as a can of baked beans or a couple of poached eggs. Others are more imaginative for the adventurous!

Do not butter toast or spread it with any other fat unless the recipe indicates that you should. Calories given are for butter, but subtract 50 calories for each ½oz (15g) fat if you use low-fat spread.

RED BEEF

Calories 250; Fibre 8g

¼ bunch watercress
1oz (25g) cooked lean beef, thinly sliced
2 teaspoons tomato chutney
2oz (55g) cooked beetroot, sliced

Cover the toast with the watercress; cut the beef into thin shreds and mix with the chutney. Pile on to the watercress and garnish with beetroot.

CREAMY MUSHROOMS

Calories 250; Fibre 9g

4oz (115g) button mushrooms
4fl oz (115ml) skimmed milk
2 teaspoons cornflour
1 tablespoon low-fat natural yogurt

salt and pepper
a dash of Worcestershire sauce

Poach the mushrooms in the milk for 5 minutes. Blend the cornflour with a little cold water and stir into the mushrooms. Bring to the boil, stirring, and cook for 2 minutes until thickened. Add the yogurt, seasoning to taste and Worcestershire sauce. Serve on toast.

BANANA SPECIAL

Calories 275; Fibre 12g

1 banana (6oz, 170g)
2 teaspoons lemon juice
a little grated lemon rind
a small fresh peach (4oz, 115g)
ground cinnamon

Mash the banana with the lemon juice and rind, and spread over toast. Peel and slice the peach, arrange on the banana and sprinkle lightly with cinnamon.
    Other fruit in season can replace the peach; melon, for instance.

DEVILLED KIDNEY

Calories 300; Fibre 6g

$\frac{1}{4}$oz (7g) butter
5oz (140g) sliced lamb's kidneys
1oz (25g) onion, chopped
salt and pepper
4 teaspoons made mustard
2 teaspoons tomato ketchup
2 large lettuce leaves
parsley for garnish

Melt the butter in a non-stick pan and fry the kidneys and onion. Off the heat add the seasonings, mustard and ketchup, and stir well. Cover the toast with the lettuce leaves. Pile the kidneys on top and sprinkle with parsley.

TOMATO BONANZA

Calories 300; Fibre 9g

½oz (15g) butter
2 teaspoons fresh basil, chopped, *or* 1 teaspoon dried basil
8oz (225g) tomatoes, thinly sliced
salt and pepper

Mix the butter and herbs together and spread over the toast. Arrange tomatoes on top, making sure the toast is completely covered. Season. Grill until the tomatoes are cooked.

CHINESE VEGETABLE TOP

Calories 300; Fibre 10g

1 large Chinese leaf
½ tablespoon oil
1 clove garlic, crushed
2oz (55g) mushrooms, thinly sliced
2oz (55g) leek, thinly sliced
2oz (55g) courgettes, thinly sliced
½ teaspoon soy sauce
1 tablespoon stock, wine, cider or water
pepper

Put half a Chinese leaf on each slice of toast. Heat the oil, add the vegetables and fry quickly for 3 minutes. Add the soy sauce, liquid and pepper. Cook for a further minute and then pile on to the leaves and serve.

HOT INDIAN CHICKEN

Calories 325; Fibre 6g

2oz (55g) curd cheese
¼–½ teaspoon curry or vindaloo paste
2oz (55g) cooked chicken, sliced
1 teaspoon mango chutney
coriander leaves or parsley

Mix curd cheese and curry paste, and spread over the toast. Arrange the chicken slices on top. Put chutney in centre of each and garnish with the leaves.

TUNA MIX

Calories 325; Fibre 7g

3½oz (100g) can tuna in brine, drained
1 medium onion, peeled
1 tablespoon Hellman's Reduced Calorie Lemon Mayonnaise
1 tablespoon chopped parsley
cayenne pepper
parsley

Flake the tuna. Cut the onion into halves and then into very thin slices. Mix with mayonnaise, parsley and pepper. Spread on toast. Garnish with parsley sprigs.

SMOKED MACKEREL SPREAD

Calories 325; Fibre 7g

2oz (55g) curd cheese
1oz (25g) smoked or kippered mackerel, flaked
pepper
2oz (55g) tomato
2 black olives

Mix the curd cheese and mackerel until smooth. Season with pepper and spread on toast. Thinly slice the tomato and olives and arrange on top.

COTTAGE CHEESE AND PINEAPPLE

Calories 325; Fibre 7g

4oz (115g) cottage cheese (natural or with onion and peppers)
salt and pepper
2 slices canned pineapple in natural juice, drained
sprigs of watercress

Season the cottage cheese to taste and spread over the toast. Top each with a ring of pineapple and heat through under the grill. Garnish with watercress.

MUSHROOM SCRAMBLE

Calories 325; Fibre 7g

2fl oz (55ml) skimmed milk
2oz (55g) mushrooms, sliced
2 eggs (size 4)
salt and pepper

Put the milk and mushrooms in a saucepan. Heat gently for 3 minutes. Beat the eggs with the seasoning and stir into the mushrooms. Cook, stirring continuously until the eggs are creamy. Serve on toast.

CRANBERRY TONGUE TREAT

Calories 350; Fibre 6g

½oz (15g) cranberry sauce
2oz (55g) tongue
1in (2·5cm) unpeeled cucumber

Spread the sauce on toast. Cut the tongue into strips and pile on top. Cut the cucumber into small dice and scatter over the tongue.

DUTCH CHEESE SAVOURY

Calories 350; Fibre 7g

2oz (55g) Edam cheese, grated
1 tablespoon horseradish sauce
2 pickled onions, thinly sliced
paprika

Mix the cheese and sauce, spread on toast and, if wished, grill until the cheese melts. Garnish with onions and paprika. Serve hot or cold.

MOCK PIZZA

Calories 350; Fibre 8g

2 small or 1 large tomato, sliced
salt and pepper
$\frac{1}{4}$ teaspoon dried mixed herbs
2oz (55g) Edam cheese, grated
2 stuffed olives, sliced

Cover the toast with the sliced tomatoes. Season to taste and sprinkle over the herbs. Top with the grated cheese and add the slices of olive for garnish. Grill until the cheese is melted.

LEMON AND PEAR SWEETENER

Calories 350; Fibre 9g

$2\frac{1}{2}$oz (70g)
1 tablespoon lemon curd
1 small ripe pear
$\frac{1}{2}$oz (15g) raisins

Mix the cottage cheese and lemon curd and spread over toast. Halve the pear, remove the core and slice thinly. Arrange on toast, sprinkle with raisins and serve at once.

BAKED BEAN MEDLEY

Calories 350; Fibre 22g

8oz (225g) baked beans with tomato sauce
2 tablespoons low-fat natural yogurt
salt and pepper
2 teaspoons chopped mint
2 lettuce leaves, shredded
a few beansprouts (optional)

Mash the baked beans and stir in the remaining ingredients. Spread on toast. If wished, arrange a few beansprouts in the centre of each.

BAKED BEANS

Calories 350; Fibre 22g

8oz (225g) baked beans with tomato sauce

Heat and serve on toast.

APPLE AND CHEESE

Calories 375; Fibre 9g

2 tablespoons sweet pickle
4oz (115g) eating apple, cored and thinly sliced
2 processed cheese slices

Spread each piece of toast with pickle and cover with sliced apple. Arrange a cheese slice on top of each and grill until the cheese has melted.

CORN, CELERY AND CHEESE GRILL

Calories 375; Fibre 14g

half a 12oz (340g) can sweetcorn
salt and pepper
2 sticks celery
1oz (25g) Lancashire cheese
paprika
2 cocktail gherkins

Liquidize the corn and its liquid and season. Slice the celery thinly and cut the cheese into small dice. Arrange the celery on toast, coat with the sweetcorn, scatter the cheese on top and grill until the cheese melts and browns. Sprinkle with paprika and garnish each with a gherkin fan.

SWEETCORN SCRAMBLE

Calories 375; Fibre 11g

2 tablespoons (30ml) skimmed milk
2 eggs (size 4)
salt and pepper
3oz (85g) canned sweetcorn, drained
1 teaspoon chopped fresh parsley

Beat the milk, eggs and seasoning together. Pour into a non-stick pan and stir in the sweetcorn. Heat gently, stirring continuously, until the egg is just set. Spoon on to toast and sprinkle with the chopped parsley.

CHICKEN LIVER SAVOURY

Calories 400; Fibre 6g

4oz (115g) chicken livers
salt and pepper
¼ teaspoon butter
2 tablespoons low-calorie tartare sauce
½oz (15g) grated carrot
2 pieces celery leaf

Put livers on foil, season and flake butter on top. Grill until lightly cooked, turning once. Meanwhile spread toast with tartare sauce and cover with carrot. Slice livers and arrange on top. Garnish with the celery leaf or a sprig of any suitable herb.

EGG, PEA AND HAM

Calories 400; Fibre 9g

2 small eggs, size 5
1½oz (40g) frozen peas
1 tablespoon low-fat natural yogurt
salt and pepper
1oz (25g) lean cooked ham, shredded

Hard-boil eggs, cook peas and chop together while hot. Stir in yogurt and seasonings. Spread on toast, make a border with the ham and serve at once.

GLAZED PEANUT AND APPLE

Calories 400; Fibre 10g

2 teaspoons crunchy peanut butter
2 teaspoons redcurrant jelly
1 teaspoon lemon, orange or other unsweetened fruit juice
1 unpeeled, small crisp apple, quartered and cored

Spread peanut butter over toast. Soften the jelly in the fruit juice over a low heat. Slice the apple thinly and stir into the jelly until the slices are coated. Arrange the apple on butter, pour any remaining jelly on top and leave for few minutes to set.

MEXICAN SPREAD

Calories 400; Fibre 13g

2oz (55g) Mattesson's Liver & Bacon Spreading Pâté
half a 10oz (283g) can red kidney beans, drained
½ stick celery, thinly sliced
1 small tomato, chopped
4 drops tabasco or pepper sauce

Chop pâté and put into a pan with the other ingredients. Heat very gently, stirring until blended and hot. Spread over toast.

DATE AND ORANGE TOPPING

Calories 400; Fibre 14g

2oz (55g) dried dates
2 small oranges
¼oz (7g) flaked almonds

Stew the dates with the juice of 1 orange and beat smooth. Cool; spread on toast. Top with the second orange, divided into segments, and scatter the almonds on top.

POACHED EGGS

Calories 425; Fibre 6g

2 medium eggs, size 3, poached without fat
½oz (15g) butter

Serve poached eggs on buttered toast.

CRUNCH CAMEMBERT

Calories 425; Fibre 7g

2oz (55g) Camembert cheese
½oz (15g) dry roasted peanuts, chopped
cayenne pepper
sprigs of watercress

Slice the Camembert very thinly and cover the toast with cheese. Sprinkle the peanuts on top and press into cheese. Grill until the cheese melts and then sprinkle with a pinch of cayenne and garnish with watercress sprigs.

SEAFOOD TOPS

Calories 425; Fibre 7g

1½oz (40g) taramasalata
6 small green pepper rings
2oz (55g) peeled prawns

Spread the toast with taramasalata. Arrange 3 pepper rings overlapping, diagonally, on each. Divide the prawns between the rings.

SCRAMBLED EGG AND KIPPER

Calories 450; Fibre 6g

2oz (55g) skinned kipper fillet
2 small eggs, size 5
salt and pepper
1 tablespoon skimmed milk
¼oz (7g) butter
2 large lettuce leaves
4 thin slices cucumber

Cut the kipper fillets into strips. Beat the eggs with the seasonings and milk. Melt the butter in a non-stick pan and pour in all but 1 tablespoon of the egg mixture; stir over moderate heat until just set. Stir in the remaining egg. Put a lettuce leaf on each toast; divide the egg between them. Arrange the kipper strips on top and decorate each with two cucumber twists. Serve at once, hot or cold.

SANDWICH SECTION

Wholemeal bread, as everyone knows, is a good source of dietary fibre. So a sandwich made from wholemeal bread makes a quick and satisfying little meal.

Those who eat a desk lunch might carry one of these sandwiches with them to work, with the two pieces of fruit allowed on the daily eating plan. At home, a sandwich might suit the housewife who wants to save most of her calories and culinary effort for the evening.

We have divided the sandwiches into three sections: simple sandwiches, for those who like to keep to old favourites; sandwiches for those who like to experiment a little; and toasted sandwiches.

Important: all the sandwiches, in both sections, must be made with two slices of wholemeal bread weighing no more than 2½oz (70g) in total. This provides you with 6g dietary fibre and 150 calories. These figures, along with the sandwich filling, are included when we list the calorie and fibre total for each sandwich. Make sure the bread is wholemeal – not just brown!

Very important: do not butter the bread, or spread even with low-fat spreads, unless this is indicated in the instructions.

SIMPLE SANDWICHES

COTTAGE CHEESE AND CUCUMBER

Calories 200; Fibre 6g

2oz (55g) cottage cheese (natural, with chives, with onions and peppers, or with pineapple)
1oz (25g) cucumber, sliced

Fill the bread with the cottage cheese and cucumber slices.

SARDINE AND TOMATO

Calories 225; Fibre 7g

1 teaspoon low-fat spread
1 sardine in tomato sauce
a dash of vinegar
1 tomato, sliced
salt and pepper

Spread one slice of the bread with the low-fat spread. Mash the sardine with the vinegar and spread on the bread. Cover with the tomato slices. Season to taste and top with the second slice of bread.

CHICKEN AND CORN RELISH

Calories 225; Fibre 7g

1¼oz (35g) pot minced chicken in jelly
1 tablespoon corn relish

Spread the bread with the minced chicken and the corn relish.

BEEF, ONION AND TOMATO

Calories 225; Fibre 7g

1¼oz (35g) pot beef paste
1 tablespoon chopped onion
1 small tomato, sliced
salt and pepper

Spread both slices of bread with the beef paste and fill with the chopped onion and sliced tomato. Season to taste.

PRAWN AND SALAD SANDWICH

Calories 225; Fibre 7g

1 tablespoon low-calorie salad dressing
1oz (25g) prawns
1 lettuce leaf
1 tomato, sliced
a few slices of cucumber
a few sprigs of watercress

Spread both slices of bread with the salad dressing and fill with the remaining ingredients.

EGG AND CRESS

Calories 250; Fibre 6g

1 tablespoon Waistline Low-Calorie Vegetable Spread
1 egg (size 3), hard-boiled and chopped
½ carton mustard and cress
salt and pepper

Spread the bread with the low-calorie vegetable spread. Fill with the egg and cress, and season to taste.

CORNED BEEF AND PICKLE

Calories 250; Fibre 6g

1 level teaspoon low-fat spread
1oz (25g) corned beef
1 tablespoon sweet pickle

Spread the bread with the low-fat spread. Fill with the corned beef and pickle.

CHEESE AND PICCALILLI

Calories 250; Fibre 7g

1oz (25g) Edam cheese, grated
1oz (25g) piccalilli, chopped finely

Mix the cheese with the piccalilli and use to fill the sandwich.

PEANUT BUTTER

Calories 325; Fibre 8g

1oz (25g) peanut butter
½ carton mustard and cress

Spread the bread with the peanut butter and fill with the mustard and cress.

SOMETHING-DIFFERENT SANDWICHES

Note: use wholemeal bread (2½oz, 70g, for two slices) as in the previous section.

COTTAGE CHEESE AND MUSHROOMS

Calories 175; Fibre 7g

1oz (25g) cottage cheese
a pinch of mixed dried herbs
2oz (55g) mushrooms, thinly sliced

Mix the cottage cheese with the herbs and spread over one slice of bread, then add the mushrooms and top with the second slice of bread.

SOFT CHEESE AND PRUNES

Calories 225; Fibre 10g

1oz (25g) Sainsbury's Low Fat Soft Cheese
1oz (25g) prunes, stoned and chopped.

Combine the cheese and prunes and fill the bread.

COTTAGE CHEESE, CAPER, SWEETCORN AND OLIVES

Calories 225; Fibre 9g

1oz (25g) cottage cheese
6 capers, drained and chopped
1oz (25g) sweetcorn
½oz (15g) olives, stoned and chopped

Mix all the ingredients together and season with pepper and mild paprika. Spread on one slice of bread and top with second slice.

PEANUT BUTTER AND BEANSPROUTS

Calories 250; Fibre 8g

½oz (15g) peanut butter
1oz (25g) beansprouts

Rinse, drain and chop the beansprouts. Spread one slice of bread with peanut butter; add the beansprouts and the second slice of bread.

PEANUT BUTTER, WATERCRESS AND MUSHROOMS

Calories 250; Fibre 9g

½oz (15g) peanut butter
1 tablespoon watercress, chopped
2oz (55g) mushrooms, finely chopped
1 teaspoon lemon juice

Spread the bread with the peanut butter. Mix the watercress, mushrooms and lemon juice together and use to fill the sandwich.

COTTAGE CHEESE, HAM AND SWEETCORN

Calories 250; Fibre 8g

1 oz (25g) cottage cheese
1 teaspoon French mustard
1oz (25g) sweetcorn
1oz (25g) lean ham

Mix the cottage cheese with the mustard and corn, and spread it over one slice of bread. Top with the ham and the second slice of bread.

EGG, COTTAGE CHEESE AND RED PEPPER

Calories 250; Fibre 7g

1oz (25g) cottage cheese
1 canned red pepper, well drained and chopped
1 egg (size 4), hard-boiled and chopped
salt and pepper
2 drops tabasco sauce

Mash together the cottage cheese, red pepper and egg. Season with salt, pepper and tabasco sauce and fill the sandwich.

CRAB AND BEANSPROUTS

Calories 275; Fibre 7g

½oz (15g) Primula or Dairylea cheese spread
1½oz (40g) canned crab meat
1oz (25g) beansprouts, chopped

Spread the cheese on the bread. Flake the crab meat, mix it with the beansprouts and fill the sandwich with it.

CRAB AND MUSHROOM

Calories 275, Fibre 6g

1 teaspoon low-fat spread
2oz (55g) canned crab meat, drained
1 tablespoon low-calorie salad dressing
1oz (25g) mushrooms, chopped

Spread the bread with the low-fat spread. Flake the crab meat and mix with the dressing and mushrooms. Fill the sandwich.

PEANUT BUTTER AND CHICKEN

Calories 300; Fibre 7g

½oz (15g) peanut butter
1oz (25g) lean roast chicken

Spread one slice of bread with the peanut butter. Top with the chicken and the second slice of bread.

BANANA, HONEY AND RAISINS

Calories 300; Fibre 11g

1 medium banana (6oz, 170g)
2 teaspoons honey
1oz (25g) raisins

Peel and mash the banana with the honey and raisins. Spread the bread with the mixture.

PEANUT BUTTER AND PRAWNS

Calories 300; Fibre 7g

½oz (15g) peanut butter
2oz (55g) prawns
thin slices of cucumber

Spread the bread with the peanut butter, and fill with the prawns and cucumber.

PEANUT BUTTER AND RAISINS

Calories 300; Fibre 9g

½oz (15g) peanut butter
1oz (25g) raisins

Mix together the peanut butter and raisins and spread on one slice of bread. Top with the second slice.

DATE AND NUT

Calories 325; Fibre 9g

1oz (25g) Sainsbury's Low Fat Soft Cheese
1oz (25g) dates, washed, dried and chopped
½oz (15g) peanuts, chopped

Spread the cheese on one slice of bread; sprinkle the nuts and dates over the surface. Top with the second slice of bread.

TURKEY AND APPLE

Calories 325; Fibre 8g

½oz (15g) cheese spread
2oz (55g) roast turkey
5oz (140g) apple, cored and thinly sliced
1 teaspoon lemon juice

Spread the cheese on the bread. Fill with the turkey and the apple slices, sprinkled with lemon juice.

TOASTED SANDWICHES

MUSHROOM AND HAM

Calories 300; Fibre 11g

half 7½oz (213g) can Chesswood Sliced Large Mushrooms in Brine
1oz (28g) boiled ham, lean only
1 tablespoon (15ml) tomato ketchup or brown sauce
½ carton mustard and cress

Drain the mushrooms. Chop the ham and mix with the mushrooms and tomato ketchup or brown sauce to make the filling. Toast the two slices of bread on one side only. Spread the filling between the toasted sides of bread. Toast the sandwich on the outside. Cut into four and garnish with mustard and cress.

DATE AND CHEESE

Calories 375; Fibre 14g

1oz (28g) stoned dates
1oz (28g) curd cheese
4oz (115g) eating apple, cored and cut into wedges

Chop the dates finely and mix with the curd cheese. Toast the two slices of bread on one side only. Spread the date and cheese filling between the two toasted sides of bread. Toast the sandwich on the outside. Cut into four and serve with the wedges of apple.

SWEETCORN AND CHICKEN

Calories 375; Fibre 12g

2oz (56g) canned sweetcorn kernels, drained
2oz (56g) cooked chicken, finely chopped
1 tablespoon (15ml) low-calorie salad cream

salt and pepper
$\frac{1}{2}$ carton mustard and cress

Mix the sweetcorn kernels, chopped chicken and low-calorie salad cream together to make the filling. Season to taste. Toast the two slices of bread on one side only. Spread the filling between the toasted sides of bread. Toast the sandwich on the outside. Cut into four and serve with mustard and cress.

ADDING FRUIT TO YOUR DAILY MENU

Two items of fruit, an apple or pear plus an orange (to ensure Vitamin C), are included as a basic part of your F-Plan menu. However, there is no reason why you should not add extra fruit as long as it is included in your total daily calorie allowance. In the case of fresh fruit this can be an easy way to add extra fibre at a modest cost in calories. Raspberries and blackberries when in season (or bought frozen) are unbeatable sources of low-calorie dietary fibre.

The chart gives close approximate calorie values of the most popular fruits in easy-to-add figures and the fibre supplied in each case.

With dried fruit, eaten neat, you have to be more restrained as the calorie count is higher. We have listed calories and grams of fibre per ounce of these dried fruits.

Fruit	Quantity	Calories	Fibre (g)
Raspberries	4oz (115g)	30	8
Blackberries	4oz (115g)	30	8
Fresh figs	2½oz (70g), one whole fruit	30	2
Strawberries	4oz (115g)	30	3
Peach	4 oz (115g), one medium-sized fruit	35	1
Plums	4oz (115g)	40	2
Orange	6oz (170g), one medium-sized fruit	40	3
Pears	5oz (140g), one medium-sized fruit	40	2
Apple	5oz (140g), one medium-sized fruit	50	2
Cherries	4oz (115g)	50	2
White grapes	4oz (115g)	70	1
Banana	6oz (170g), one medium-sized fruit	80	3
Dried fruit			
Prunes	1oz (25g) raw weight	45	4

Fruit	Quantity	Calories	Fibre (g)
Apricots	1oz (25g) raw weight	55	6
Dried figs	1oz (25g) raw weight	60	5
Dried dates (weighed with stones)	1oz (25g)	60	2
Sultanas	1oz (25g) raw weight	70	2
Raisins	1oz (25g) raw weight	70	2
Dried dates (weighed without stones)	1oz (25g)	70	3

HI-FI YOGURT DESSERTS

BLACKBERRY YOGURT

Calories 100; Fibre 4g

5oz (140g) low-fat natural yogurt
2oz (55g) blackberries
Liquid or powdered artificial sweetener (optional)

Stew the blackberries with a tablespoon water until just tender. Sweeten to taste with liquid or powdered artificial sweetener, if liked, then cool. Stir the yogurt into the cooled stewed blackberries and serve.

RASPBERRY YOGURT

Calories 125; Fibre 4g

2oz (55g) raspberries, fresh, or frozen and thawed
2 teaspoons icing sugar
5oz (140g) low-fat natural yogurt

Crush the raspberries with the icing sugar, then stir into the yogurt and chill before serving.

PEAR AND HAZELNUT YOGURT

Calories 150; Fibre 3g

5oz (140g) low-fat natural yogurt
5oz (140g) eating pear, cored and chopped
6 shelled hazelnuts, chopped

Mix the yogurt with the chopped pear and hazelnuts and serve.

HONEY BRAN AND SULTANA YOGURT

Calories 150; Fibre 4g

½oz (15g) Allinson's Honey Bran
½oz (15g) sultanas
5oz (140g) low-fat natural yogurt

Stir the Honey Bran and sultanas into the yogurt and serve.

APPLE AND RAISIN YOGURT

Calories 175; Fibre 3g

5oz (140g) low-fat natural yogurt
5oz (140g) eating apple, cored and chopped
½oz (15g) raisins
1 walnut half, chopped

Mix the yogurt with the chopped apple, raisins and walnut.

RAISIN AND BRAN YOGURT

Calories 175; Fibre 3g

1oz (25g) raisins, chopped
3 tablespoons unsweetened or fresh orange juice
5oz (140g) low-fat natural yogurt
1 tablespoon bran

Soak the raisins in the orange juice for ½ hour, then stir in the yogurt and bran.

BANANA AND WALNUT YOGURT

Calories 175; Fibre 4g

6oz (170g) banana, peeled and sliced
1 walnut half, chopped
5oz (140g) low-fat natural yogurt

Stir the sliced banana and chopped walnut into the yogurt and serve.

PRUNE YOGURT

Calories 175; Fibre 8g

2oz (55g) dried prunes *or*
  4oz (115g) cooked prunes (unsweetened)
1 tablespoon unsweetened orange juice
5oz (140g) low-fat natural yogurt

If using dried prunes, either cover with cold water and soak overnight
or cover with boiling water and soak for 1 hour, then bring to the boil,
cover and simmer for 15–20 minutes. Drain and cool. Halve the cooked
prunes and remove stones. Stir the prunes and orange juice into the
yogurt. Chill and serve.

ORANGE AND COCONUT YOGURT

Calories 200; Fibre 5g

5oz (140g) low-fat natural yogurt
5oz (140g) orange, segmented
½oz (15g) desiccated coconut

Mix the yogurt with the orange segments and coconut. Leave to stand
for ½ hour before serving to allow the flavours to blend.

APRICOT YOGURT

Calories 200; Fibre 9g

5oz (140g) low-fat natural yogurt
2oz (55g) dried apricots, chopped
1 teaspoon liquid honey

Mix the yogurt and chopped apricots together and leave to stand for a minimum of 12 hours for the apricots to soften. Stir in the honey just before serving.

BLACKCURRANTS WITH YOGURT AND BISCUITS

Calories 275; Fibre 8g

half 10·6oz (300g) can Ribena Blackcurrants in Syrup
2 tablespoons (30ml) low-fat natural yogurt
2 Country Basket Six Grains or Yogurt Biscuits

Mix the canned blackcurrants with the yogurt and serve with the biscuits.

APPLE AND DATE DESSERT BAR AND YOGURT

Calories 250; Fibres 6g

5·3oz (150g) carton low-fat natural yogurt
1 level teaspoon (5ml) liquid honey
2 level tablespoons ($\frac{1}{4}$oz/7g) Meadow Farm Toasted Bran
1 Prewett's Apple and Date Dessert Bar

Spoon the yogurt into a dish. Stir in the honey and sprinkle the top with the toasted bran. Serve with the apple and date dessert bar.

HI-FI BAKED APPLES

Baked apples make ideal low-calorie, high-fibre desserts or snack meals. The different fillings help to ring the changes and enable you to serve baked apples frequently without boredom creeping in.

BAKED APPLE – BASIC RECIPE

Calories 60; Fibre 5g

8oz (225g) cooking apple
filling as given in recipes

Wash the apple and remove the core, leaving a hole for filling. Cut through the skin round the centre of the apple with a sharp knife to prevent it bursting during cooking. Place the apple in a small ovenproof dish and pour 2–4 tablespoons water round the apple. Cover with a lid or foil and bake at 350°F (180°C, gas 4) for 30–40 minutes or until the apple is tender right through but not overcooked. Serve hot or cold.

Note: Some fillings are added after the apple is baked and some are added before baking. Each recipe will indicate at which stage the filling is added.

BAKED APPLE WITH BLACKBERRIES

Calories 100; Fibre 13g .

8oz (225g) cooking apple
4oz (115g) blackberries
1 teaspoon sugar
liquid sweetener to taste (optional)

Prepare the apple for baking (see above). Pack 1oz (25g) blackberries into core hole of apple. Pour 2–4 tablespoons water around the apple. Cover with a lid or foil and bake at 350°F (180°C, gas 4) for 30 minutes or until apple is cooked through. Cook the remaining blackberries in a little water until tender, then stir in the sugar. Mash the blackberries with a fork or purée in an electric blender, and sweeten to taste with liquid sweetener, if wished. Serve baked apple with the hot blackberry sauce poured over.

BAKED APPLE WITH ORANGE AND CHERRY

Calories 125; Fibre 6g

8oz (225g) cooking apple
4oz (115g) orange
1 teaspoon honey
1 glacé cherry, quartered

Bake the apple without stuffing (see opposite). Meanwhile grate a little rind from the orange. Halve the orange – squeeze the juice from one half and remove the segments from the other half. Heat the orange juice with the honey in a small pan. Off the heat add the orange segments, grated rind and glacé cherry. Spoon into the centre of the baked apple.

MINCEMEAT STUFFED BAKED APPLE

Calories 125; Fibre 6g

8oz (225g) cooking apple
1oz (25g) mincemeat

Fill the centre of the apple with the mincemeat. Bake (see opposite). Serve hot.

BAKED APPLE WITH APRICOT AND CINNAMON

Calories 125; Fibre 9g

1oz (25g) dried apricots
2 tablespoons unsweetened orange juice
8oz (225g) cooking apple
a pinch of ground cinnamon

Chop the apricots and place in a small basin or cup with the orange juice. Leave to stand overnight. Sprinkle the cut surface on the inside of the apple with ground cinnamon. Spoon in the apricots and any remaining juice. Bake (see p. 196). Serve hot.

DATE AND HONEY STUFFED BAKED APPLE

Calories 150; Fibre 7g

1oz (25g) stoned dates, chopped
1 teaspoon clear honey
8oz (225g) cooking apple

Mix the chopped dates with the honey and spoon into the centre of the apple. Bake (see p. 196). Serve hot.

FRUIT AND NUT STUFFED BAKED APPLE

Calories 175; Fibre 6g

8oz (225g) cooking apple
½oz (15g) mixed raisins and sultanas
1 tablespoon unsweetened orange juice
½oz (15g) chopped mixed nuts

Bake the apple without stuffing (see p. 196). Meanwhile soak the raisins and sultanas in the orange juice for 30 minutes. Mix with the nuts and spoon into the centre of the baked apple. Serve hot.

BAKED APPLE WITH BANANA AND WALNUT

Calories 175; Fibre 8g

8oz (225g) cooking apple
1 small banana (about 5oz, 140g)
1 tablespoon low-fat natural yogurt
¼oz (7g) walnut pieces

Bake the apple without stuffing (see p. 196). Mash the banana until soft and stir in the yogurt and walnut pieces. Spoon into the centre of the hot baked apple and serve.

STEWED FRUIT DESSERTS

In this section you will find mostly simple stewed fruit desserts. For some stewed fruits variations have been given where appropriate.

We have used a little sugar to sweeten those fruits which we feel require sweetening; however, if you prefer to save calories by using a non-sugar sweetener, you can subtract 16 calories for each level teaspoon of sugar replaced. (Remember that where a spoonful of sugar is indicated this always means a *level* spoonful.)

STEWED BLACKBERRIES

Calories 50; Fibre 8g

4oz (115g) blackberries
1 level teaspoon granulated sugar

Stew the blackberries with 2 tablespoons water in a covered pan until softened. Stir in the sugar.

STEWED PEAR

Calories 75; Fibre 2g

a 5oz (140g) dessert pear
1 teaspoon lemon juice
a strip of lemon rind
a pinch of ground cinnamon
2 teaspoons granulated sugar

Peel, halve and core the pear. Place the pear halves in a pan with the lemon juice, lemon rind, cinnamon, sugar and 2½fl oz (70ml) water. Cover and simmer until the pear is tender but not mushy. Lift out the pear halves and boil the liquid rapidly until reduced by half. Discard the lemon rind. Pour the liquid over the stewed pears. Serve hot or cold.

STEWED RHUBARB

Calories 75; Fibre 3g

4oz (115g) rhubarb
2 tablespoons unsweetened orange juice
a pinch of ground ginger
½oz (15g) granulated sugar

Cut the rhubarb into 1in (2·5cm) lengths and place in a small pan with the orange juice, ginger and sugar. Cover and simmer until the rhubarb is just tender. Serve hot or cold.

STEWED GOOSEBERRIES

Calories 75; Fibre 4g

4oz (115g) gooseberries
1 elderflower head, if available
½oz (15g) granulated sugar

Stew the gooseberries with 2 tablespoons water and the elderflower head, if used, in a covered saucepan, until just tender. Remove the elderflower head and stir in the sugar.

STEWED BLACKBERRIES AND APPLE

Calories 75; Fibre 6g

2oz (55g) blackberries
4oz (115g) cooking apple, peeled, cored and sliced
1½ teaspoons granulated sugar

Stew the blackberries and apple with 2 tablespoons water in a covered pan until the fruits are tender. Stir in the sugar.

STEWED BLACKCURRANTS

Calories 75; Fibre 10g

4oz (115g) blackcurrants
1 sprig mint
2½ teaspoons granulated sugar

Stew the blackcurrants with 2 tablespoons water and the mint in a covered pan until softened. Stir in the sugar.

STEWED PLUMS WITH ALMONDS

Calories 100; Fibre 3g

4oz (115g) Victoria plums
2½fl oz (70ml) unsweetened orange juice
¼oz (7g) flaked almonds

Stew the plums in the orange juice until just tender. Serve hot or chilled, topped with the flaked almonds.

STEWED APPLE

Calories 100; Fibre 4g

8oz (225g) cooking apple, peeled, cored and sliced
a strip of lemon rind
2 cloves
2½ teaspoons granulated sugar

Put the apple, lemon rind and cloves with 2 tablespoons water in a pan and simmer, covered, until the apple is softened. Remove the lemon rind and cloves and stir in the sugar. Serve hot or cold.

RHUBARB AND BANANA

Calories 150; Fibre 6g

5oz (140g) banana, sliced
1 portion stewed rhubarb
1 walnut half, chopped

Mix the sliced banana with the rhubarb and top with the chopped walnut.

STEWED PRUNES

Calories 100; Fibre 8g

2oz (55g) dried prunes
water or cold tea to cover
4 drops angostura bitters
a strip of lemon peel
½ teaspoon sugar

Cover the prunes with cold water or strained tea and leave to stand overnight. Place the prunes and soaking liquid in a pan and add the angostura bitters and lemon peel. Cover and simmer for 20 minutes. Remove the lemon peel, stir in the sugar and serve hot or cold.

STEWED DRIED FIGS

Calories 125; Fibre 10g

2oz (55g) dried figs
a strip of lemon rind

Cover the figs with water and soak overnight. Turn the figs and liquid into a pan, add the lemon rind and cover and simmer for about 40 minutes, until the figs are tender. Serve hot or cold.

STEWED DRIED APRICOTS

Calories 125; Fibre 14g

2oz (55g) dried apricots
4 tablespoons unsweetened orange juice

Put the dried apricots in a bowl with the orange juice and water to cover and leave to soak overnight. Turn the apricots and soaking liquid into a pan and simmer, covered, for 30 minutes or until the apricots are tender. Serve hot or cold.

APPLE WITH SULTANAS AND NUTS

Calories 150; Fibre 6g

a pinch of ground cinnamon
½oz (15g) sultanas
8oz (225g) cooking apple, stewed as above
1 walnut half, chopped

Stir the cinnamon and sultanas into the apple and heat gently for 2 minutes. Serve topped with the chopped walnut.

APPLE WITH ORANGE

Calories 150; Fibre 6g

8oz (225g) cooking apple, stewed as above
4oz (115g) orange, peeled and segmented
1 glacé cherry

Allow the stewed apple to become cold. Stir in the orange segments and decorate with the glacé cherry.

STEWED PRUNES WITH BANANA

Calories 150; Fibre 11g

1 small banana (4½oz, 115g), sliced
1 portion stewed prunes, without sugar

Add the sliced banana to the hot or cold stewed prunes and serve.

STEWED PEAR IN RED WINE WITH FLAKED ALMONDS

Calories 150; Fibre 3g

a 5oz (140g) dessert pear
a strip of lemon rind
2½fl oz (70ml) red wine
2 teaspoons soft brown sugar
¼oz (7g) flaked almonds

Peel the pear and leave whole. Place in a small pan with the lemon rind, red wine and brown sugar. Cover and simmer on one side until tender. Turn the pear over and cover and simmer until the other side is tender. Stand the pear upright in a serving dish and stick the flaked almonds in it. Pour the cooking liquid round it and serve.

DRIED FRUIT SALAD

Calories 150; Fibre 13g

3oz (85g) mixed dried fruit (prunes, apricots, peaches and pears)
2 tablespoons concentrated low-calorie orange squash
¼ teaspoon ground cinnamon

Put the fruit, orange squash and water to cover the fruit in a bowl and leave to soak overnight. Place fruit and liquid in a pan, add cinnamon, cover and simmer for 30–40 minutes, until tender. Serve hot or cold.

SOME SAMPLE MENUS

Here, and on the following pages, you will see some examples of the many ways in which F-Plan meals can be put together to suit your own way of life and preferred eating pattern.

As you follow the diet you will probably – in the typical way of many slimmers – keep returning to some favourite meals which you learn off by heart. But do try to keep sampling some new dishes as well, from the very wide selection in this book, to keep your diet interesting and nutritious.

1,000 CALORIE MENU

The kind of meal selection which would suit a busy working girl, taking her lunch to work and cooking something quick and easy for her evening meal.

	Calories	Fibre (g)
Daily allowances: Fibre-Filler, ½ pint skimmed milk, two items of fruit	400	20
Breakfast Half portion of Fibre-Filler with milk from allowance		
Office lunch Cottage cheese, ham and sweetcorn sandwich (p. 185); apple and orange from allowance	250	8
Evening meal Frankfurter bean bake (p. 135)	350	16
Suppertime snack Remaining portion of Fibre-Filler		
TOTAL	1,000	44

1,000 CALORIE MENU

A 'little and often' meal selection for the housewife at home with a tendency to eat frequent snacks.

	Calories	Fibre (g)
Daily allowances: Fibre-Filler, ½ pint (3dl) skimmed milk, two items of fruit	400	20
Mid-morning Late breakfast on half portion of Fibre-Filler with milk from allowance		
Lunch Sweetcorn chowder with wholemeal bread (p. 162); orange from allowance	200	6
Teatime Remaining portion of Fibre-Filler; an apple from allowance		
Evening meal Creamy mushrooms on toast (p. 168)	250	9
Suppertime snack Fruit, veg and cheese on crispbread (p. 166)	150	7
TOTAL	1,000	42

1,250 CALORIE MENU

The meals on this menu are particularly quick and easy to make.

	Calories	Fibre (g)
Daily allowances: Fibre-Filler, ½ pint (3dl) skimmed milk, two items of fruit	400	20

Breakfast
Half portion of Fibre-Filler with milk from allowance; an orange from allowance

Lunch

	Calories	Fibre (g)
Bacon and baked beans (p. 132); an apple or pear from allowance	275	16

Evening meal

	Calories	Fibre (g)
Apple and cheese on toast (p. 174);	375	9
orange and coconut yogurt (p. 194)	200	5

Suppertime snack
Remaining portion of Fibre-Filler

TOTAL	1,250	50

1,250 CALORIE MENU

The pattern of this menu is based on the common slimmer's preference for being 'strict' during the day – when it is often easier – and saving most calories for the hungry hours of the evening.

	Calories	Fibre (g)
Daily allowances: Fibre-Filler, ½ pint (3dl) skimmed milk, two items of fruit	400	20
Breakfast Half portion of Fibre-Filler with milk from allowance; an orange from allowance		
Lunch Prawn and pepper salad (p. 146); a pear from allowance	100	5
Late afternoon Remaining portion of Fibre-Filler to bridge the gap		
Evening meal Grilled bacon steak with baked jacket potato and baked beans (p. 101);	375	8
for dessert, mincemeant stuffed baked apple (p. 197)	125	6
Late supper Egg and cress sandwich (p. 182)	250	6
TOTAL	1,250	45

1,500 CALORIE BACHELOR MENU

No-bother meals for the man who has to make them for himself.

	Calories	Fibre (g)
Daily allowances: Fibre-Filler, ½ pint (3dl) skimmed milk, two items of fruit	400	20
Breakfast Full daily allowance of Fibre-Filler with milk from allowance; an orange from allowance		
Lunch Two peanut butter and prawn sandwiches (p. 186); an apple from allowance	600	14
Evening meal Baked chicken, jacket potato and sweetcorn (p. 103);	400	8
large (8oz, 225g) banana (figures calculated from chart on p. 286)	100	4
TOTAL	1,500	46

1,500 CALORIE DRINKING MAN'S MENU

This menu illustrates how you can allow yourself some alcohol by using the chart on p. 279.

	Calories	Fibre (g)
Daily allowances: Fibre-Filler, ½ pint (3dl) skimmed milk, two items of fruit	400	20
Breakfast Full daily allowance of Fibre-Filler with milk from allowance		
Lunch Two corned beef and pickle sandwiches (p. 182); an apple and an orange from allowance	500	12
Evening meal Pease pudding with lamb's liver (p. 129)		
Alcohol Three pub singles of whisky, gin or vodka	150	
TOTAL	1,500	42

Calorie and Fibre Charts

On the following pages you will find calorie and fibre charts which will make it easy for you to plan your own high-fibre meals if you prefer to do so rather than follow the ready-planned meal suggestions.

Instant Calorie and Fibre Guide

Is it very fattening? Is it rich in fibre? Because this chart gives the calorie and dietary fibre contents of average or easily recognizable portions of all the basic foods, it provides an instant answer to these questions.

Few of us can picture an ounce of lamb chop or an ounce of apple, pear or peach, but we do get a clear picture of an average-sized whole loin chop, or an apple, pear or peach. Are these foods costing us much in calories and what, if anything, is each one contributing to our intake of dietary fibre? The answers emerge clearly here, as do the foods which will be of greatest value in boosting our fibre intake as we follow the F-Plan method of dieting.

Only foods which are most easily recognizable on a 'per ounce' basis are listed in that form in this chart. However, as you measure your food to keep within your calorie total, your portion or piece of a particular food may be larger or smaller than the average one itemized here. For this reason we also provide a Basic Calorie and Fibre Chart, starting on page 285, which reveals the calories and dietary fibre in a single ounce of each of the foods listed here.

In this guide we list only very basic packaged foods like cornflakes. But these days, with a growing awareness of the value of dietary fibre for health and weight control, many manufacturers are packaging useful fibre-rich foods. Some other canned, frozen and packaged foods just happen to be useful sources of dietary fibre because of the nature of their contents. You will find our valuable Calorie and Fibre Guide to Packaged Foods on page 242.

In this next chart, calorie figures are rounded off to the nearest 5, and fibre figures to the nearest half gram, for easy calculation. Dietary fibre figures should always be considered as an approximate rather than a precise guide. The figures we give are sufficiently dependable to take your daily intake up to the right level to help reduce your weight and protect your health.

Use the Instant Calorie and Fibre Chart to check which foods are low enough in calories to help you keep within your total and high enough in fibre to help you to reach that daily target.

Instant Calorie and Fibre Chart

Food	Portion	Calories	Fibre g
All Bran	1½oz (42g), average breakfast bowl	105	11·5
Almonds	1 shelled almond	10	0·5
ground	1 level tablespoon (15ml)	30	1·0
Apples			
eating	5oz (142g), average-sized fruit	50	2·0
cooking			
baked	8oz (227g), average-sized baking apple	70	4·5
stewed without sugar	6oz (170g)	55	3·5
Apricots			
fresh			
weighed with stone	1oz (28g), average-sized fruit	5	0·5
stoned and stewed without sugar	6oz (170g)	40	3·0
dried, stewed without sugar	4oz (113g) cooked weight	75	10.0
dried, raw	1oz (28g)	50	6.5
canned	4oz (113g), fruit and syrup	120	1.5

Food	Portion	Calories	Fibre g
Arrowroot	1 level teaspoon (5ml)	10	0
Asparagus, boiled	1 spear	5	0·5
Aubergines, raw, flesh only	1 aubergine, 7oz (200g)	30	5·0
Avocado, flesh only	½ avocado, 3½oz (99g)	215	2.0
Bacon	1 bacon steak, grilled, 3½oz (99g) raw weight	105	0
	1 back rasher		
	raw	150	0
	grilled	85	0
	fried	95	0
	1 streaky rasher		
	raw	85	0
	grilled	60	0
	fried	70	0
Banana	6oz (110g), average-sized fruit	80	3·5
Barcelona nuts, shelled	1oz (28g)	180	3·0

Barley, pearl	½oz (14g) raw weight, amount in average portion of thick broth	50	1·0
Bean sprouts			
raw	2oz (56g), average salad portion	15	0·5
cooked	2oz (56g)	20	0·5
Beans			
adzuki, uncooked	1oz (28g) dry weight	90	7·0
baked, canned in tomato sauce	8oz (227g), one small can	145	16·5
black-eyed, uncooked	1oz (28g) dry weight	95	7·0
broad, boiled	4oz (113g)	50	5·0
butter, canned	4oz (113g) drained weight	110	5·5
french, boiled	4oz (113g)	10	3·5
haricot, uncooked	1oz (28g) dry weight	75	7·0
red kidney			
uncooked	1oz (28g) dry weight, usual portion in a dish like chilli con carne	75	7·0
boiled	3oz (85g), average portion in salad	75	7·0
canned	3oz (85g) drained weight, average portion in a dish like chilli con carne	75	7·0
runner, boiled	4oz (113g)	20	4·0
soya, uncooked	1oz (28g) dry weight	110	4·0

Food	Portion	Calories	Fibre g
Beef			
beefburgers, frozen	average 2oz (56g) beefburger		
	grilled	130	0
	well grilled	85	0
brisket, boiled	3oz (85g)	275	0
corned, canned	2oz (56g)	120	0
forerib, roast	3oz (85g), lean only	190	0
mince, stewed	3oz (85g)	180	0
rump steak, grilled	4oz (113g), lean only	190	0
silverside, salted, boiled	3oz (85g), lean only	145	0
sirloin, roast	3oz (85g), lean only	160	0
stewing steak, stewed	3oz (85g)	185	0
topside, roast	3oz (85g), lean only	130	0
Beef sausages	1 large sausage, grilled	130	0
	1 small sausage (chipolata), grilled	60	0
Beef and pork sausages	1 large sausage, grilled	135	0
	1 small sausage (chipolata), grilled	65	0
Beetroot, boiled	2oz (56g)	25	1·5
Bemax (wheatgerm)	¼oz (7g), 1 level tablespoon (15ml)	25	0·5

Biscuits, *see* Packaged Food Chart			
Black pudding, fried	2oz (56g)	170	0·5
Blackberries, stewed without sugar	4oz (113g)	30	7·0
Blackcurrants, stewed without sugar	4oz (113g)	30	8·5
Bran	$\frac{1}{4}$oz (7g), $2\frac{1}{4}$ level tablespoons (37ml)	15	3·0
Brawn	2oz (56g)	85	0
Brazil nuts	1 shelled brazil nut	20	0·5
Bread (*see also* p. 131 for individual manufacturers' breads)			
brown	$2\frac{1}{2}$oz (70g), two average slices	155	3·5
wheatgerm (e.g. Hovis)	2oz (56g), two average slices	130	2·5
white	$2\frac{1}{2}$oz (70g), two average slices	160	2·0
wholemeal	$2\frac{1}{2}$oz (70g), two average slices	150	6·0

Food	Portion	Calories	Fibre g
Bread rolls			
brown			
crusty	2oz (56g), average size	160	3·5
soft	2oz (56g), average size	170	3·0
white			
crusty	2oz (56g), average size	160	2·0
soft	2oz (56g), average size	170	1·5
wholemeal (e.g. Allinson)	1½oz (42g), average size	90	3·5
Broccoli tops, boiled	4oz (113g)	20	4·5
Brussels sprouts, boiled	4oz (113g)	20	3·0
Butter	½oz (14g), average daily allowance on a calorie-controlled diet	105	0
Cabbage			
red, raw	1oz (28g), average serving of pickled cabbage	5	1·0
savoy, boiled	4oz (113g)	10	3·0
spring, boiled	4oz (113g)	10	2·5
white, raw	3oz (85g), average portion in coleslaw	20	2·5
winter, boiled	4oz (113g)	15	3·0

Cake			
fruit	2oz (56g), average slice	200	1·5
plain	1oz (28g), 1 small slice	100	1·0
rich, iced			
sponge, with fat, jam-filled	2oz (56g), 1 average slice	170	0·5
Carrots			
raw	2oz (56g), 1 medium-sized whole carrot	10	1·5
boiled	4oz (113g)	20	3·5
canned	4oz (113g) drained weight	20	4·0
Cashew nuts	1oz (28g)	150	0·5
Cauliflower			
raw	2oz (56g), average amount in a salad	10	1·0
boiled	4oz (113g)	10	2·0
Celeriac, boiled	4oz (113g)	15	5·5
Celery			
raw	2oz (56g), 1 large stick	5	1·0
boiled	4oz (113g)	5	2·5
Cherries			
eating	4oz (113g)	45	1·5
glacé	1 cherry	10	0

Food	Portion	Calories	Fibre g
Chestnuts, shelled	1oz (28g)	50	2·0
Chicken			
roast	3oz (85g), meat only, no skin	125	0
drumstick, grilled	3½oz (99g) weight before cooking	90	0
Chicken joint, baked or grilled	8oz (227g) weight before cooking	180	0
Chicory, raw	1oz (28g), salad serving	3	0·5
Chinese leaves, raw	2oz (56g), salad serving	5	1·0
Chips, fried in deep fat	4oz (113g), small portion	280	2·0
Chocolate, drinking	2 rounded teaspoons (20ml)	40	0
Christmas pudding	2oz (56g), small portion	170	1·0
Cocoa powder	1 rounded teaspoon (10ml)	20	0
Coconut, fresh	1oz (28g)	100	4·0
Cod			
fillet, fresh, steamed or poached	6oz (170g) weight before cooking	125	0
steak, frozen, raw	4oz (113g)	80	0

Food	Measure	Calories	Fibre
Coffee, instant, powder or granules	1 rounded teaspoon (10ml)	0	0
Coffee and chicory essence	1 teaspoon (5ml)	10	0
Coley, raw	6oz (170g)	120	0
Condensed milk, whole, sweetened	1 tablespoon (15ml)	50	0
Corn oil	1 tablespoon (15ml)	125	0
Corned beef	2oz (56g)	120	0
Cornflakes	1oz (28g), average breakfast bowl	105	0·8
Cornflour	1 level tablespoon (15ml)	35	0·5
Cottage cheese	4oz (113g) carton	110	0
Crab, canned	1½oz (42g) can	60	0
Cream	1 tablespoon (15ml) double	60	0
	1 tablespoon (15ml) single	30	0
Crispbreads, *see* p. 130 for individual manufacturers' crispbreads			
Crisps, potato	0.88oz (25g), 1 small packet	130	3·0

Food	Portion	Calories	Fibre g
Cucumber	2oz (56g), salad serving	5	0
Currants, dried	½oz (14g)	35	1·0
Custard powder	1 level tablespoon (15ml)	35	0·5
Damsons, stewed without sugar	4oz (113g)	30	3·5
Dates, dried, stoneless	2oz (56g)	140	5·0
Egg, whole, raw, boiled or poached in water	size 1	95	0
	size 2	90	0
	size 3	80	0
	size 4	75	0
	size 5	70	0
	size 6	60	0
Egg white	1 white of size 3 egg	15	0
Egg yolk	1 yolk of size 3 egg	65	0
Eggplant, *see* **Aubergines**			

Endive, raw	2 oz (56g), salad serving	5	1·0
Evaporated milk, whole	1 tablespoon (15ml)	25	0
Figs			
fresh, raw	1oz (28g), average-sized fruit	10	0·5
dried	2oz (56g) dry weight, about three dried figs	120	10·5
dried, stewed without sugar	4oz (113g)	130	11·5
Fish fingers, frozen	1 fish finger, grilled without fat	50	0
Flour, *see* Your Basic Calorie and Fibre Chart			
Fruit salad, canned	4oz (113g) fruit and juice	110	1·0
Glacé cherries, *see under* **Cherries**			
Golden syrup	1 tablespoon (15ml)	60	0
Goose, roast	3oz (85g), meat only	265	0
Gooseberries			
ripe, raw	2oz (56g)	20	2·0
stewed without sugar	4oz (113g)	15	3·0

Food	Portion	Calories	Fibre g
Grapefruit			
whole	5oz (142g), half average-sized fruit	15	0·5
canned in natural juice	4oz (113g)	45	0·5
Grapenuts	1½oz (42g), average breakfast bowl	150	3·0
Grapes			
black	4oz (113g)	55	0·5
white (green)	4oz (113g)	70	1·0
Greengages, stewed without sugar	4oz (113g)	45	2·5
Guavas, canned	4oz (113g)	70	4·0
Haddock			
fillets, fresh	6oz (170g) raw weight	120	0
smoked, steamed	6oz (170g) cooked weight	170	0
Ham			
boiled	2oz (56g), lean only	95	0
cooked and vacuum-packed	2oz (56g), 2–3 slices	80	0
canned	3oz (85g), salad serving	100	0

Food	Description	Calories	Fibre
Hazelnuts	1oz (28g) shelled weight	105	1·5
Heart, lamb's, roast	4oz (113g), average-sized heart	270	0
Herring, grilled	5oz (142g), whole herring weighed raw after head and bones removed	280	0
Honey	1 level teaspoon (5ml)	15	0
Ice cream	2oz (56g)	95	0
Jam	1 level teaspoon (5ml)	15	0
Jelly, made up with water	4oz (113g)	70	0
Kidney			
lamb	2oz (56g), average raw weight	50	0
ox	2oz (56g), average portion in a steak-and-kidney casserole	50	0
Kipper, grilled	6oz (170g), whole kipper weighed before cooking	280	0

Food	Portion	Calories	Fibre g
Lamb			
breast, roast	4oz (113g), lean and fat, no bone	460	0
leg, roast	3oz (85g), lean only	162	0
loin chops, grilled	5oz (142g), average-sized chop, raw weight	310	0
shoulder, roast	3oz (85g), lean only	165	0
Lard	½oz (14g)	125	0
Leeks, boiled	4oz (113g)	30	4·0
Lemon sole, fried coated in crumbs	4oz (113g), average-sized fish	190	0·5
Lentils, uncooked	1½oz (42g), in portion of soup	125	5·0
Lettuce, raw	1oz (28g), salad serving	5	0·5
Liver			
calf	4oz (113g) raw weight, average serving for grilling	170	0
chicken	2oz (56g) raw weights, average amount in chicken liver pâté or for fried livers on toast	75	0

Food	Serving	Calories	Fibre
lamb	4oz (113g) raw weight, average casserole serving	200	0
Liver sausage	1oz (28g), sufficient for one round of sandwiches	85	0
Loganberries			
stewed without sugar	4oz (113g)	15	6·5
canned in syrup	4oz (113g), fruit and syrup	110	3·5
Low-fat spread (e.g. Outline, St Ivel Gold)	1oz (28g), average daily allowance in a calorie-controlled diet	105	0
Luncheon meat, canned	2oz (56g)	175	0
Lychees, canned	4oz (113g), fruit and syrup	75	0·5
Macaroni, wholewheat	2oz (56g) dry weight	195	5·5
Mackerel			
whole, raw	8oz (227g)	320	0
smoked	6oz (170g)	420	0
Mandarin oranges, canned in syrup	4oz (113g), fruit and syrup	65	0·5

Food	Portion	Calories	Fibre g
Mangoes, canned	4oz (113g), fruit and syrup	90	1·0
Margarine, all brands	½oz (14g), usual daily allowance in a calorie-controlled diet	105	0
Marmalade	1 level teaspoon (5ml)	15	0
Marrow, boiled	4oz (113g)	10	1·0
Marzipan	½oz (14g)	60	1·0
Mayonnaise	1 tablespoon (15ml)	95	0
Melon cantaloup, honeydew or yellow	8oz (227g), average slice with skin	30	1·0
ogen	12oz (340g), average whole melon	60	2·5
water	8oz (227g), average slice with skin	25	1·0
Milk, dried, skimmed	1 rounded teaspoon (10ml), average serving in tea or coffee	10	0
Mincemeat	½oz (14g), average weight in a mince pie	35	0·5
Muesli, base mixture	2oz (56g), average breakfast bowl	205	4·0

Food	Serving	Calories	Fibre
Mulberries	4oz (113g) raw weight	40	2·0
Mushrooms	4oz (113g) raw weight	15	3·0
Mustard and cress	¼oz (7g), salad or sandwich serving	1	0
Nectarines	5oz (142g), average-sized whole fruit	65	3·0
Oatcakes	1oz (28g)	125	1·0
Oatmeal	1oz (28g) raw weight, to make average bowl of porridge	110	2·0
Olive oil	1 tablespoon (15ml)	125	0
Onion boiled	4oz (113g)	15	1·5
raw	½oz (14g), salad serving	5	0
Orange, whole	6oz (170g), average-sized fruit	40	2·5
Parsley	½oz (14g)	5	1·5
Parsnips, boiled	4oz (113g)	65	3·0

Food	Portion	Calories	Fibre g
Passion fruit, raw	3oz (85g), average-sized fruit	10	5·5
Pawpaw, canned	4oz (113g)	70	0·5
Peach, whole	4oz (113g), average-sized fruit	35	1·5
Peaches, canned	4oz (113g), fruit and syrup	95	1·0
Peanuts, shelled	1oz (28g)	160	2·5
Peanut butter	½oz (14g), sufficient for one sandwich	88	1·0
Pearl barley, *see* **Barley, pearl**			
Pear, whole	5oz (142g), average-sized fruit	40	2·5
Pears, canned	4oz (113g), fruit and syrup	90	2·0
Peas			
fresh, raw	1oz (28g), salad serving	20	1·5
fresh or frozen, boiled	4oz (113g) raw weight	60	9·0
garden, canned	3½oz (99g), half the drained contents of a 10oz (283g) can	45	6·0
processed, canned	3½oz (99g)	75	7·5

	Calories	Fibre
dried, uncooked		
split 1½oz (42g), in average portion of pea soup	120	7·0
2oz (56g) dry weight, amount in average portion pease pudding	175	6·5
chick		
raw 1oz (28g) dry weight	90	4·0
boiled 3oz (85g) cooked weight	90	5·0
Pepper, green		
raw 1oz (28g), salad serving	5	0·5
cooked 5oz (142g), average-sized pepper	20	1·5
Piccalilli 1oz (28g), 1 rounded tablespoon (30ml)	10	0·5
Pickle, sweet 1oz (28g), 1 rounded tablespoon (30ml)	40	0·5
Pilchards, canned in tomato sauce 2½oz (70g), average-sized pilchard	85	0
Pineapple		
fresh 2oz (56g), average slice without skin and core	25	0·5
canned in syrup 4oz (113g), fruit and syrup	90	1·0

Food	Portion	Calories	Fibre g
Plaice, fillets, fried in crumbs	6oz (170g) raw weight	435	1·0
Plums			
Victoria, dessert	2½oz (70g), average-sized fruit	15	1·5
cooking, stewed without sugar, weighed with stones	6oz (170g)	40	3·5
Pork			
chop, grilled	7oz (200g) raw weight, fat cut off after grilling	315	0
leg, roast	3oz (85g), lean only	155	0
Pork sausages, grilled	2oz (56g), large sausage, raw weight	135	0
	1oz (28g), 1 chipolata, raw weight	65	0
Porridge	1oz (28g), oatmeal or porridge oats made up with water	110	2·0
Potato			
baked	7oz (200g), eaten with skin	170	5·0
roast	2oz (56g)	90	1·0
instant, mashed	1oz (28g) dry weight	90	4·5

		Calories	Fibre
old, boiled and mashed	4oz (113g)	90	1·0
new			
boiled	4oz (113g)	85	2·5
canned	4oz (113g) drained weight	60	3·0
Prawns, shelled	2oz (56g)	60	0
Prunes, dried			
with stones	1oz (28g), four to five prunes	38	3·8
stewed without sugar	4oz (113g) cooked weight	85	8·5
Puffed wheat	¾oz (21g), average breakfast bowl	70	3·5
Rabbit, stewed	6oz (170g), weighed on the bone	150	0
Radishes, raw	1oz (28g), salad serving	5	0·5
Raisins	½oz (14g), serving with cereal etc.	35	1·0
Raspberries			
raw	4oz (113g)	30	8·5
canned in syrup	4oz (113g), fruit and syrup	95	5·5
Redcurrants, stewed without sugar	4oz (113g)	20	8·0

Food	Portion	Calories	Fibre g
Rhubarb	4oz (113g) raw weight	10	3·0
Rice Krispies	1oz (28g), average breakfast bowl	105	1·0
Rice			
brown	2oz (56g) dry weight, usual amount for a rice-based meal	200	2·5
white	2oz (56g) dry weight	205	1·5
Rock salmon, fried in batter	6oz (170g)	445	0·5
· **Sago**	½oz (14g) raw weight, usual amount in a serving of milk pudding	50	0·5
Salad cream	1 level tablespoon (15ml)	50	0
Salad dressing, low-calorie (e.g. Waistline, Heinz)	1 level tablespoon (15ml)	25	0
Salami	1oz (28g)	135	0
Salmon, canned	3oz (85g) drained weight	170	0
Salsify, boiled	4oz (113g)	20	1·0

		Calories	Fibre
Sardines			
canned in oil	2oz (56g), weighed after draining off oil	120	0
canned in tomato sauce	2oz (56g)	100	0
Scampi, in breadcrumbs, fried	3oz (85g)	265	1·0
Sea-kale, boiled	4oz (113g)	10	1·0
Semolina	½oz (14g) dry weight, amount in a serving of milk pudding	50	0·5
Shortcrust pastry			
white flour, cooked	1½oz (42g), usual amount in a serving of flan	220	1·0
wholemeal flour, cooked	1½oz (42g)	210	3·0
Shredded Wheat	¾oz (21g), one Shredded Wheat	70	2·5
Spaghetti			
white	2oz (56g), dry weight, usual amount in a pasta dish	210	1·5
brown wholewheat	2oz (56g) dry weight	195	5·5
canned in tomato sauce	7oz (200g), half large can	120	2·0
Spinach, boiled	4oz (113g)	30	7·0

Food	Portion	Calories	Fibre g
Spring greens, boiled	4oz (113g)	10	4·5
Spring onions	½oz (14g), salad serving	5	0·5
Strawberries, raw	4oz (113g)	30	2·5
Sugar	1 rounded teaspoon (10ml)	35	0
Sugar Puffs	1oz (28g), average breakfast bowl	95	1·5
Sultanas	½oz (14g), serving with cereal etc.	35	1·0
Sunflower seeds	¼oz (7g), just a nibble	35	0·5
Swedes, boiled	4oz (113g)	20	3·0
Sweetcorn kernels, canned	3½oz (99g)	75	5·5
Syrup, golden	1 level tablespoon (15ml)	60	0
Tangerine	3oz (85g), average-sized fruit	60	1·0
Tapioca	½oz (14g) dry weight, usual amount in a serving of milk pudding	50	0·5

Tomatoes			
fresh	4oz (113g), two, average-sized	15	1·5
canned	4oz (113g)	10	1·0
Tongue, ox, pickled, boiled	2oz (56g)	165	0
Treacle, black	1 level tablespoon (15ml)	50	0
Tripe, stewed	6oz (170g)	170	0
Trout	6oz (170g) raw weight	150	0
Tuna			
canned in brine	7oz (198g) can	230	0
canned in oil	7oz (198g) can	365	0
Turnips, boiled	4oz (113g)	15	2·5
Turkey, roast	3oz (85g), meat only, no skin	115	0
Veal			
cutlet, coated in egg and breadcrumbs, fried	3oz (85g)	180	0
fillet, roast	3oz (85g)	190	0
Vegetable oil	1 level tablespoon (15ml)	125	0

Food	Portion	Calories	Fibre g
Walnuts	1oz (28g) shelled weight	145	1·5
Watercress	1oz (28g), generous salad serving	5	1·0
Weetabix	two biscuits	115	4·5
Wheatgerm	½oz (15g), 1 rounded tablespoon (30ml)	45	0·5
Whitecurrants, stewed without sugar	4oz (113g)	25	6·5
Yogurt, low-fat			
natural	5·3oz (150g) carton	80	0
flavoured	5·3oz (150g) carton	120	0
hazelnut	5·3oz (150g) carton	160	2·5

Calorie and Fibre Guide to Packaged Foods

Here, available to the public for the first time, is a comprehensive guide to the useful fibre-supplying packaged foods.

Dietary fibre is not an easy substance to measure, and in order to reveal this valuable information we have had to draw on the assistance of the manufacturers themselves in some cases, and in others on the help of the technicians at London University and the analytical experts working for Dr David Southgate at the Food Research Institute.

It is important to emphasize that the values given for fibre are approximate. Fibre-measuring methods are still in their infancy. Different brands and packages of the same type of food will differ a little in their precise composition. But the figures here will provide you with a good enough guide to ensure that you reach that 30-grams-plus daily fibre total to ease and speed your slimming and help protect your health.

The quantities given in this guide are those which we feel will be most convenient to you in planning your menus. Usually we list the number of calories and the amount of dietary fibre in a whole can or package. From the weight of the can or package you will easily be able to assess whether this is an individual portion or multi-portion pack.

In the case of some foods we felt that other measures would help you more. The fibre content of different breads, for instance, is given on a per-ounce basis. Slices and sizes vary so much that it makes most sense to weigh your own average slice of your own chosen loaf to reveal the calories and fibre in that. With biscuits, the calories and dietary fibre in one or two whole biscuits is obviously of more instant value than that in a whole package. Throughout this guide we have used this kind of commonsense flexibility to make calorie- and fibre-counting easy for you.

The same principle has been applied in 'rounding off' calorie and fibre figures for easy calculation. Where the contents of a whole pack are given we round off to the nearest 5 calories and half-gram of fibre, which gives a close enough guide.

In selecting and rejecting the foods to be included in this guide we have been equally realistic. All canned fruits, for instance, will provide at least a little dietary fibre. However, with some the fibre quantity is small in relation to the calorie cost. For this reason we have listed only the canned fruits which are free of added sugar, apart from those, like raspberries and prunes, which are particularly rich sources of dietary fibre.

Canned and packaged foods can play a valuable role in modern weight-conscious and health-conscious eating – when you use the information in this guide.

Ready packaged foods can help to provide an alternative. One of the remarkable effects of the F-Plan diet is the major influence it has already had on the sales pattern of foods in Britain, signalling a major upswing in the consumption of foods like wholewheat and granary bread, bran, and bran cereals.

Britain is at last beginning to eat in the way that our medical and nutritional advisers have been urging us to eat – and, quick to spot the trend, manufacturers already have new fibre-rich foods in the pipeline which are likely to start appearing in the shops soon. So, with the aid of these and the fibre figures revealed for the first time in this book, it becomes easier and easier to shed weight and improve health with the F-Plan.

Calorie and Fibre Chart of Packaged Foods

	Calories	*Fibre g*

Biscuits

	Calories	Fibre g
Bran biscuits, per biscuit		
Allinson		
Bran Biscuit	78	1·0
Bran Oatcake	39	1·0
Boots Second Nature Bran	44	1·3
Country Basket Wholewheat		
Bran	32	1·7
Crawfords Bran Oatcake	50	1·3
Fox's		
Wholemeal Bran	67	1·0
Bran Crunch	32	0·4
Holly Mill Natural Bran	33	0·8
R. M. Scott Husky Wholemeal		
Bran	37	0·2
St Michael Wholemeal Bran	65	1·0
Coconut biscuits, per biscuit		
Allinson Coconut	70	0·9
Fox's Coconut Cookies	74	0·8
Digestive biscuits, per biscuit		
Burton's Digestive Sweetmeal,		
from 200g pack	47	0·5
Hovis Digestive	56	0·7
Huntley & Palmer Digestive	63	0·5
McVitie Digestive Wheatmeal,		
from 400g pack	70	0·8
Mitchelhill's Digestive	63	0·1
Sainsbury's Sweetmeal Digestive,		
from 400g pack	60	0·5
Tesco Digestive, from 250g pack	65	0·8

	Calories	*Fibre g*
Fig biscuits, per biscuit		
Jacob's Fig Roll	53	0·7
Prewett's Fig	60	0·7
Fruit and/or nut biscuits, per biscuit		
Allinson		
Carob-coated Fruit & Nut	62	0·2
Fruit & Nut	77	0·6
Hazelnut	63	0·5
Peanut	61	0·4
Walnut	65	0·5
Boots		
Second Nature Wholemeal Fruit Bran	33	1·1
Second Nature Wholemeal Hazelnut	37	0·5
Country Basket Hazelnut	34	1·2
Fox's Oat & Fruit	77	0·6
Garibaldi biscuits, per biscuit		
Peak Frean Garibaldi	30	0·3
Muesli-type biscuits, per biscuit		
Allinson Muesli	61	0·7
Boots Second Nature Wholemeal Muesli Fruit	38	0·4
Country Basket Muesli Fruit	37	1·0
Fox's Muesli Finger	63	0·7
Oatmeal and oatflake biscuits, per biscuit		
Allinson		
Oatmeal	74	0·4
Bran Oatcake	39	1·0
Carob-coated Oatmeal	62	0·2
Country Basket Oatmeal	34	1·6
Crawford's Bran Oatcake	50	1·3

	Calories	Fibre g
Fox's		
Oaten Crunch	36	0·3
Oatflake Cookie	69	0·4
Oat & Fruit Biscuit	77	0·6
Paterson's		
Girdle Oatcake	50	0·5
Farmhouse Oatcake	90	0·8
Shortbread, per piece		
Allinson Wholemeal Shortbread	82	1·2
Wheaten biscuits, per biscuit		
Fox's Wheaten Cookies	69	0·5
Prewett's Wholemeal	65	0·4
Miscellaneous biscuits, per biscuit		
Allinson		
Carob-coated Ginger/Bran	61	0·4
Demerara	66	0·4
Ginger	49	0·6
Honey	57	0·7
Boots Second Nature Wholemeal		
Six Grains	37	0·4
Country Basket		
Six Grains	34	1·5
Yogurt	34	1·2
Fox's		
Fivers	85	0·8
Nice	39	0·3
Itona Granny Ann High Fibre	100	5·0
Jacob's Farmhouse	34	0·4
Mitchelhill's Healthy Life	61	0·1
Prewett's		
Carob Chip Cookies	65	0·4
Sesame & Sunflower Cookies	67	0·5
Stem Ginger Cookies	59	0·4

	Calories	*Fibre g*
Crispbreads and crackers, per biscuit		
Country Basket Wholewheat		
Crispbread	32	0·7
Crisp-i-Bran	19	2·9
Energen		
Brancrisp	23	1·3
Starch Reduced Bran	18	0·7
Starch Reduced Brown Wheat	17	0·4
Starch Reduced Cheese	19	0·3
Starch Reduced Rye	17	0·4
Starch Reduced Wheat	18	0·2
Jacob's		
Vitawheat	28	0·7
Vitawheat, Rye	28	0·7
Parkstone Bakeries Crackerbread	23	0·3
Primula Extra Thin	20	0·1
Ryvita		
Brown	25	0·9
Original	25	0·9
Salt-free	25	0·9

Brans

	Calories	*Fibre g*
Soya brans, per oz (28g)		
Direct Foods Soya Bran	24	9·9
Granose Soya Bran	60	9·9

	Calories	*Fibre g*
Wheat brans, per oz (28g)		
Allinson		
Bran Plus	63	7·1
Broad Bran	43	12·5
Boots Second Nature Natural		
Unprocessed Bran	56	12·4
Itona Wheat Bran	43	12·5
Prewett's Natural Wheat Bran	43	12·5

	Calories	Fibre g

Breads

Bran loaves, per oz (28g)

Nimble Family Bran	70	1.3
Sunblest Hi Bran	57	3·1
Sunblest Sunbran	62	1·3
Windmill Bran	64	1·8

Granary, per oz (28g)

Windmill Granary	67	1·6

Wheatgerm loaves, per oz (28g)

Hovis

Family Loaf	63	1·4
Handy Loaf	66	1·4
Original	66	1·4
Vitbe Wheatgerm	65	1·4

Wheatmeal (brown) loaves, per oz (28g)

Mothers Pride Brown Long Loaf	64	1·6
Windmill Country Brown	64	1·6

White loaves, per oz (28g)

Mothers Pride

Danish Toaster	71	0·9
Danish White	71	0·9
White Long Loaf	66	0·8

Nimble

Family White	71	0·9
Long White	74	0·8
Sunblest White	65	0·8
Windmill White Fibre	64	1·7

Wholemeal loaves, per oz (28g)

Allinson Wholemeal	61	2·4

Windmill

Wholemeal, small loaf, 400g	64	2·6
Wholemeal, large loaf, 800g	61	2·4

	Calories	*Fibre g*
Bread rolls, per oz (28g)		
Granose Wheatmeal Rolls	100	1·0
Granose White Rolls	101	0·5
Bread mixes, per packet dry mix		
Allinson		
Bran Bread Mix, 1¼lb pack	2,050	75·0
Wholewheat Bread Mix, 1¼lb pack	1,845	57·0
Prewett's Ever-ready Bread Mix,		
1¼lb pack	1,895	48·0

Breakfast Cereals

	Calories	*Fibre g*
Maize (corn) breakfast cereals, per oz (28g)		
Cornflakes, *see* Your Basic Calorie and Fibre Chart		
Kellogg's		
Crunchy Nut Corn Flakes	107	0·5
Frosties	100	0·3
Muesli-type and crunchy breakfast cereals,		
per oz (28g) except where stated		
Boots		
Second Nature Honey Muesli	118	2·2
Second Nature Muesli	103	2·1
Cheshire		
Wholefoods Muesli	104	0·8
Wholefoods Economy Muesli	93	0·5
Familia		
Birchermuesli	115	2·0
Muesli (Swiss Mixed Cereal),		
1 portion pack, 2½oz (71g)	285	5·5
Holly Mill		
Muesli	103	1·8
Muesli Base	101	2·1
Sugar Free Muesli	98	2·0
Jordans		
Country Muesli	103	0·7
Muesli Tub, Banana and Brazil,		
2½oz (71g) tub	305	3·6

	Calories	Fibre g
Muesli Tub, Coconut and Sultana, 2½oz (71g) tub	260	3·6
Muesli Tub, Date and Cashew, 2½oz (71g) tub	263	3·6
Original Crunchy Natural	123	0·4
Original Crunchy with Honey, Almonds and Raisins	121	0·4
Original Crunchy with Bran and Apple	116	0·7
Kellogg's Country Store	100	1·4
Prewett's		
Bran Muesli	87	6·2
Honey Muesli	104	1·8
Muesli Base	105	2·1
Muesli Deluxe	111	2·1
Muesli	102	1·9
Quaker		
Harvest Crunch	126	2·6
Harvest Crunch, Bran & Apple	129	3·9
Safeway Swiss Style Breakfast Cereal	110	2·0
Sainsbury's Swiss Style Breakfast Cereal	100	2·0
Sunwheel Natural Foods Fruit and Nut Muesli	103	3·0
Tesco Swiss Style Breakfast Cereal	105	2·0
Weetabix Alpen	105	1·9
Oat breakfast cereals, per oz (28g)		
Boots Second Nature Bran & Oat Crunch	103	5·4
Lyons Tetley		
Ready Brek, Butter Flavour	110	2·2
Ready Brek, Standard Flavour	110	2·2
Prewett's		
Breakfast Oats	115	2·0
Oatmeal, fine/medium/coarse	115	2·0
Porridge, wheatmeal	95	2·7

	Calories	Fibre g
Oat breakfast cereals, *cont.*		
Quaker		
Golden Oaties	107	2·3
Oats	105	4·3
Oat Krunchies	108	3·4
Warm Start	107	4·3
Safeway		
Hot Oat Cereal	115	2·2
Quick Cooking Oats	105	4·0
Sainsbury's Scotch Porridge		
Oats	105	4·0
Scotts Porage Oats	115	4·0
Tesco		
Instant Oats	115	2·2
Scotch Porridge Oats	115	4·0
Waitrose Instant Porridge	115	2·2
Whitworth's Porridge Oats	114	2·0
Rice breakfast cereals, per oz (28g)		
Kellogg's		
Rice Krispies	99	0·3
Ricicles	100	0·3
Coco Pops	101	0·3
Puffa Puffa Rice	117	0·1
Wheat (including bran) breakfast cereals, per oz (28g) except where stated		
Allinson Crunchy Bran	64	7·7
Boots Second Nature Bran & Oat		
Crunch	103	5·4
Energen		
Brancrunch	115	4·3
Wheatflakes	100	4·2
Granose		
Fruit Bran	86	3·5
Sunnybisk, each	50	1·1
Holly Mill Wheat-Heart	117	1·0

	Calories	Fibre g
Kellogg's		
All-Bran	70	8·0
Bran Buds	74	7·4
Bran Flakes	85	4·2
Sultana Bran	82	3·6
Smacks	106	0·2
Meadow Farm Toasted Bran	100	8·2
Nabisco		
Bran Flakes	105	3·4
Shredded Wheat, each	80	2·4
Shreddies	105	2·3
Spoonsize	100	3·1
Prewett's Whole Wheat Flakes	102	2·6
Quaker		
Puffed Wheat	106	4·3
Sugar Puffs	104	2·1
Safeway Biskwheat, each	68	2·5
Sainsbury's		
Puffed Wheat	100	4·3
Whole Wheat Bisk, each	70	2·5
Weetabix		
Bran Fare	75	8·2
Farmhouse Bran	85	5·7
Weetabix, per biscuit	58	2·2
Weetaflakes	96	3·6
Miscellaneous breakfast cereals, per oz (28g)		
Bird's Grape-Nuts	99	2·0
Holly Mill		
Day Brek	118	5·2
Bran Brek	123	2·3
Kellogg's Special K	101	0·5
Prewett's Golden Grains	105	1·6
Pronutro	105	3·4

Chutneys and Pickles

Bicks Corn Relish, per oz (28g)	30	1·3

	Calories	Fibre g
Chutneys and Pickles, *cont.*		
Happy Farm		
Piccalilli, per oz (28g)	9	0·5
Sweet Pickle, per oz (28g)	38	0·5
Tomato & Apple Chutney, per oz (28g)	48	0·5
Dehydrated Meals		
Vesta Chilli con Carne with Rice,		
pack, serves two	800	19·0
Flour		
Rye flour, per oz (28g)		
Prewett's Rye Flour	96	0·3
Soya flour, per oz (28g)		
Prewett's Soya Flour	123	3·4
White flour (plain, self-raising and strong flours),		
per oz (28g)		
Allinson		
81% Farmhouse (plain)	100	2·3
81% Farmhouse (self-raising)	100	2·3
Strong White	97	1·1
Prewett's		
Millstone Flour 81% (plain)	97	2·3
Millstone Flour 81% (self-raising)	100	2·3
Strong White Bread Flour		
(unbleached)	97	1·1
Super White Unbleached Flour (plain)	97	1·4
Super White Unbleached Flour		
(self-raising)	97	1·1
Whitworths		
Plain White Flour	99	1·0
Self-Raising White Flour	96	1·0
Wholemeal flour		
Allinson		
100% Wholemeal Flour (plain)	96	3·1

	Calories	Fibre g
Cerea 100% Flour	96	3·1
Boots Second Nature Stoneground		
Wholemeal Flour	89	2·7
Jordans 100% Wholewheat Flour	91	0·7
Prewett's		
100% Organic Wholemeal Flour	96	3·1
100% Wholemeal Flour (plain)	96	3·1
100% Wholemeal Flour (self-raising)	96	3·1

Fruit, Canned

Apples

	Calories	Fibre g
Waitrose Apple Slices in Natural Juice,		
7¾oz (219g) can	75	4·5

Apricots

	Calories	Fibre g
Boots Shapers Apricots in Low-calorie		
Syrup, 7¾oz (220g) can	35	3·0
Dietade Apricots in Water,		
7oz (198g) can	35	2·5
Frank Cooper's Apricots in Water,		
7oz (198g) can	25	2·5
Sainsbury's Apricot Halves in Apple		
Juice, 14½oz (411g) can	185	5·5

Blackberries

	Calories	Fibre g
Sainsbury's Blackberries in Syrup,		
7½oz (213g) can	210	10·5
Smedley Blackberries in Syrup,		
7½oz (213g) can	145	10·0
Weight Watchers Blackberries in		
Low-calorie Syrup, 7oz (198g) can	50	10·0

Blackcurrants

	Calories	Fibre g
Ribena Blackcurrants in Syrup,		
300g can	345	13·0
Sainsbury's Blackcurrants in Syrup,		
7½oz (213g) can	210	9·0
Smedley Blackcurrants in Syrup,		
7½oz (213g) can	145	9·0

	Calories	Fibre g
Fruit salad		
Dietade		
Fruit Salad in Water, 7oz (198g) can	35	2·0
Fruit Salad in Fruit-sugar Syrup,		
8oz (227g) can	90	2·5
Frank Cooper's Fruit Salad in Water,		
7oz (198g) can	35	2·0
Weight Watchers Fruit Salad in		
Low-calorie Syrup, 7oz (198g) can	35	2·0
Gooseberries		
Hartley's Gooseberries,		
10oz (283g) can	240	5·5
Safeway Gooseberries, 10oz (283g) can	180	5·5
Sainsbury's Gooseberries,		
10½oz (298g) can	210	6·0
Smedley Gooseberries, 10oz (283g) can	180	5·0
Grapefruit		
John West Grapefruit Segments in		
Natural Juice, 10oz (283g) can	120	1·0
Libby's Grapefruit Segments,		
sweetened, 19oz (538g) can	380	2·0
Princes Grapefruit Segments,		
10oz (283g) can	170	1·0
Sainsbury's Grapefruit Segments in		
Natural Juice, 19oz (539g) can	210	2·0
Tesco Grapefruit Segments,		
sweetened, 19oz (539g) can	340	2·0
Waitrose Grapefruit in Natural Juice,		
7¾oz (219g) can	75	1·0
Weight Watchers Grapefruit		
Segments in Low-calorie Syrup		
7oz (198g) can	50	1·0
Loganberries		
Tesco Loganberries in Syrup,		
14½oz (411g)	320	13·5

	Calories	Fibre g
Mandarin oranges		
John West Mandarin Orange		
Segments in Natural Juice,		
10½oz (298g) can	80	1·0
Peaches		
Boots Shapers Peachers in Low-calorie		
Syrup, 7¾oz (220g) can	45	2·0
Dietade Peaches in Water, 7oz (198g) can	35	2·0
Frank Cooper's Peaches in Water,		
7oz (198g) can	35	2·0
John West Peach Slices in Fruit Juice,		
10oz (283g) can	130	3·0
Koo Peach Slices in Apple Juice,		
8oz (227g) can	95	2·5
Sainsbury's Peaches in Apple Juice,		
14½oz (411g) can	185	4·0
Waitrose Peaches in Apple Juice,		
7¾oz (219g) can	75	2·0
Weight Watchers Peaches in Low-		
calorie Syrup, 7oz (198g) can	40	2·0
Pears		
Boots Shapers Pears in Low-calorie		
Syrup, 7¾oz (220g) can	50	3·5
Dietade		
Pears in Water, 7oz (198g) can	35	3·5
Pears in Fruit-sugar Syrup,		
8oz (227g) can	95	4·0
Frank Cooper's Pears in Water,		
7oz (198g) can	35	3·5
John West Pear Quarters in Fruit		
Juice, 10oz (283g) can	110	5·0
Koo Pear Halves in Apple Juice,		
8oz (227g) can	105	4·0
Sainsbury's Pear Halves in Apple Juice,		
14½oz (411g) can	185	7·0

	Calories	Fibre g
Pears, *cont.*		
Waitrose Pears in Apple Juice, 7¾oz (219g) can	75	3·5
Weight Watchers Pears in Low-calorie Syrup, 7oz (198g) can	40	3·5
Pineapple		
Boots Shapers Pineapple in Low-calorie Syrup, 7¾oz (220g) can	55	2·0
Del Monte Pineapple Slices in Natural Juice, 8oz (227g) can	150	2·0
Dietade		
Pineapple in Water, 7oz (198g) can	35	2·0
Pineapple in Fruit-sugar Syrup, 8oz (227g) can	100	2·0
Frank Cooper's Pineapple in Water, 7oz (198g) can	40	2·0
John West Pineapple Rings in Natural Juice, 8oz (227g) can	130	2·0
Sainsbury's Pineapple Slices in Natural Juice, 8oz (227g) can	105	2·0
Waitrose Pineapple in Natural Juice, 8oz (227g) can	120	2·0
Weight Watchers Pineapple Rings in Low-calorie Syrup, 7oz (198g) can	70	2·0
Prunes		
Pickering Prunes in Syrup, 7½oz (213g) can	220	7·5
Tesco Prunes in Syrup, 7½oz (213g) can	235	9·0
Raspberries		
Baxters		
Raspberries in Syrup, 10¼oz (290g) can	250	14·5
Raspberries in Syrup, 15oz (425g) can	365	21·0

	Calories	Fibre g
Hartleys Raspberries in Syrup, 15oz (425g) can	400	21·0
Sainsbury's Raspberries in Syrup, 7½oz (213g) can	155	10·5
Smedley Raspberries in Syrup, 7½oz (213g) can	155	9·0
Weight Watchers Raspberries in Low-calorie Syrup, 7oz (198g) can	50	10·0

Strawberries
Baxters
Strawberries in Syrup, 10¼oz (290g) can	250	3·0
Strawberries in Syrup, 15oz (425g) can	365	4·0
Weight Watchers Strawberries in Low-calorie Syrup, 7oz (198g) can	50	2·0

Fruit, Dried

Whitworths
Apricots, no-need-to-soak, 8·8oz (250g)	385	52·5
Chopped Dates, sugar rolled, 8·8oz (250g)	680	17·5
Dessert Dates, with stones, 8·8oz (250g)	530	18·5
Stoned Dates, 8·8oz (250g)	620	21·5
Figs, 8·8oz (250g)	450	37·5
Prunes, no-need-to-soak, 8·8oz (250g)	290	30·0

Pasta

Wholewheat Pasta, per oz (28g)
Newform Foods Limited Country
Basket Spaghetti	99	2·3
Record
Whole Wheat Lasagne, uncooked	105	2·8

	Calories	Fibre g
Wholewheat Pasta (Record), *cont.*		
Whole Wheat Long Spaghetti, uncooked	105	2·8
Whole Wheat Short Cut Macaroni, uncooked	105	2·8
Whole Wheat Spaghetti Rings, uncooked	105	2·8

Rice

	Calories	Fibre g
Brown Rice, per oz (28g)		
Prewett's Unpolished Rice, long/short grain	97	1·4
Whitworths Brown Rice	102	0·3

	Calories	Fibre g
White Rice, per oz (28g)		
Kellogg's Boil-in-bag rice, uncooked	93	0·1
Whitworths		
Basmati Rice, uncooked	103	0·1
Ground Rice, uncooked	103	0·1
Rice, long/short grain, uncooked	103	0·1
Rice Easy Cook, uncooked	105	0·1

Savoury Pot Snacks

	Calories	Fibre g
Noodle snacks, per pot made up		
Golden Wonder		
Beef & Tomato Pot Noodle	370	1·5
Cheese & Tomato Pot Noodle	345	2·0
Chicken & Mushroom Pot Noodle	380	8·5
Spicy Curry Pot Noodle	380	4·5
Sweet & Sour Pot Noodle	345	1·0

	Calories	Fibre g
Rice snacks, per pot made up		
Golden Wonder		
Chicken Curry	265	2·5
Chicken Risotto	270	1·0

	Calories	Fibre g
Savoury Beef	255	1·5
Spicy Tomato	250	1·5

Slimmers Products

Meal replacements
Balance, per serving

(26g) with 175ml milk	198	2·0

Crunch'n'Slim

Coconut & Currant Bars, per meal	230	2·8
Orange & Raisin Bars, per meal	230	2·8
Sultana & Hazelnut Bars, per meal	230	2·8

Limits

Cheese Flavour Cracker Biscuits with Bran	250	2·5
Chocolate Biscuits with Bran	250	2·5
Chocolate Flavour Wafer with Bran	250	2·5
Chocolate Mint Biscuits with Bran	250	2·5
Coffee Flavour Biscuits with Bran	250	2·5
Lemon & Lime Flavour Biscuits with Bran	250	2·5
Milk Chocolate Sweetmeal Biscuits with Bran	250	2·5
Orange Flavour Biscuits with Bran	250	2·5
Plain Sweetmeal Digestive with Bran	250	2·5
Vanilla Flavour Biscuits with Bran	250	2·5

SlimGard, per daily quota of 1 Bar,

1 Drink and 2 Inbetweeners	333	1·7

Starch-reduced rolls

Energen Starch Reduced Rolls, each	23	0·5

Snacks

Cereal, fruit & nut bars and slices, per bar or slice
Holly Mill

Carob Chip Bar	145	0·5

	Calories	*Fibre g*
Cereal, fruit & nut bars and slices (Holly Mill), *cont.*		
Cereal & Nut Crunchy Bar	115	0·5
Crunchy Slice	185	1·0
Fruit & Nut Slice	175	1·0
Muesli Slice	215	1·0
Oat, Apple & Raisin Slice	165	1·0
Oat, Apricot & Almond Slice	175	1·0
Protein Slice	175	0·5
Roasted Peanut Bar	155	0·5
Sesame Bar	125	1·0
Jordans		
Original Crunchy Bar,		
Honey & Almond	150	0·5
Original Crunchy Bar,		
Honey & Coconut	145	1·0
Lynn Valley Wholefoods,		
Peanut & Raisin Bar	170	2·5
Prewett's		
Apple & Date Dessert Bar	120	4·0
Banana Dessert Bar	75	2·5
Date & Fig Dessert Bar	125	3·5
Fruit & Bran Bar	85	5·0
Fruit & Nut Dessert Bar	130	4·0
Muesli Fruit Bar	125	3·5
Quaker		
Harvest Crunch Bar, Almond Variety	90	1·0
Harvest Crunch Bar, Peanut Variety	90	1·0
Fruit and nut mixtures		
Cheshire Wholefoods		
Trail Pack, Fruit & Nut Mix,		
100g pack	535	5·0
Trail Pack with coconut and banana,		
56g pack	240	3·0
T. G. Smith (Liverpool) Limited		
Tropical Treat, 100g pack	410	8·0

	Calories	Fibre g
Savoury snacks		
Allinson Wheateats, per 21g packet	90	0·5

Soups

Lentil		
Baxter's Lentil, 15oz (425g) can	200	9·0
Campbell's		
Condensed Lentil, 4·9oz (140g) can,		
makes 9·8oz (280g)	130	5·5
Condensed Lentil, 10½oz (298g) can,		
makes 21oz (596g)	280	12·0
Granny Soup, Lentil,		
15oz (425g) can	240	10·0
Heinz Lentil, 10·6oz (300g) can	180	6·0
Minestrone		
Batchelor's Minestrone, packet,		
makes 1 pint	155	2·5
Crosse & Blackwell Box Soup,		
Minestrone, makes 1 pint	80	3·5
Knorr Minestrone, packet,		
makes 1½ pints	225	4·5
Sainsbury's Minestrone, packet,		
makes 1 pint	120	4·0
Pea		
Baxter's Pea & Ham, 15oz (425g)	225	10·0
Campbell's		
Condensed Pea & Ham,		
10½oz (298g) can, makes 21oz (596g)	400	13·0
Main Course Pea & Ham,		
15oz (425g) can	350	9·0
Heinz Pea & Ham, 10·6oz (300g) can	200	7·0
Vegetable		
Heinz Vegetable & Lentil Big Soup,		
15·3oz (435g) can	210	8·9

	Calories	Fibre g
Soya and Cereal Protein Foods		
Savoury mixes, per packet or can unless stated otherwise		
Brooke Bond Oxo		
Beanfeast, Bolognese, 4oz (113g) pack	330	10·0
Beanfeast, Mexican Chilli, 4oz (113g) pack	330	17·0
Beanfeast, Mild Curry, 4oz (113g) pack	320	10·0
Beanfeast, Paella Style, 4oz (113g) pack	350	13·5
Beanfeast, Soya Mince with Onion, 4oz (113g) pack	375	10·0
Beanfeast, Supreme, 4oz (113g) pack	335	13·5
Direct Foods		
Protoveg, Natural, Unflavoured, 4½oz (127g) carton	370	4·0
Protoveg, Flavoured (Beef, Ham, Pork Style), 4½oz (127g) carton	360	4·5
Protoveg Menu, Farmhouse Soya Stew Mince, 4oz (113g) carton	405	3·5
Protoveg Menu, Minced Soya & Onion Mix, 5oz (142g) carton	510	3·5
Protoveg Menu, Soya Bolognese Mix, 4oz (113g) carton	390	5·5
Protoveg Menu, Soya Mince with Vegetables, 4oz (113g) carton	395	4·0
Protoveg Menu, Burgamix, 6½oz (184g) pack	995	9·0
Protoveg Menu, Sosmix, 6½oz (184g) pack	960	5·5
Protoveg Menu, Jumbo Grills, 8oz (227g) carton	750	4·0
Protoveg Menu, Jumbo Grills Flavouring, per oz (28g)	68	0·7

	Calories	Fibre g
Protoveg Menu, Vegetable Curry, 112g pack	400	4·0
Protoveg Menu, Vegetable Goulash, 112g pack	395	3·5
Mr Fritzi Fry's Sausage Mix, 8oz (227g) pack	1,210	13·0
Mr Fritzi Fry's Savoury Mix (Burga Style), 8oz (227g) pack	1,075	8·0
Mr Fritzi Fry's Hawaiian Croquettes (Fishcake Style), 8oz (227g) pack	850	7·5
Granose		
Beef Flavour Chunks, per oz (28g) dry weight	95	0·9
Beef Flavour Mince, per oz (28g) dry weight	95	0·9
Bologna, 10oz (283g) can	475	4·0
Bologna, 15oz (425g) can	710	6·5
Bolognese Sauce, 10oz (284g) can	170	1·5
Cannelloni, 14oz (397g) can	300	1·0
Chicken Flavour Pie Filling, 10oz (284g) can	165	1·5
Goulash, 10oz (284g) can	155	1·5
Nutloaf, 15oz (425g) can	750	14·5
Nuttolene, 15oz (425g) can	1,265	14·5
Protose, 15oz (425g) can	675	14·5
Ravioli, 15oz (425g) can	270	2·5
Sausalatas, 10oz (284g) can	390	4·0
Sausalatas, 15oz (425g) can	580	6·0
Sausalene, 10oz (284g) can	555	7·5
Sausfry, per oz (28g) dry weight	140	2·6
Saviand, 10oz (284g) can	565	4·5
Savoury Cuts, 7½oz (213g) can	185	0·5
Savoury Cuts, 15oz (425g) can	375	1·0
Savoury Pudding, 11oz (312g) can	645	4·5
Savoury Pudding, Chicken Flavour, 11oz (312g) can	510	3·0

	Calories	Fibre g
Savoury mixes (Granose) *cont.*		
Soya Beans in Tomato Sauce, 7½oz (213g) can	365	7·5
Soya Beans in Tomato Sauce, 15oz (425g) can	725	15·5
Tenderbits, 7½oz (213g) can	170	0·5
Vegetable Pâté, per oz (28g)	85	1·0
Prewett's		
5 Cereal Savoury Mix, per oz (28g) dry weight	97	2·5
5 Cereal Savoury Mix, 300g pack	1,025	24·0

Spreads

	Calories	Fibre g
Sunwheel Natural Foods		
Peanut Butter, Crunchy and Smooth, per oz (28g)	169	1·4
Sesame Spread, per oz (28g)	177	1·6
Sunflower Spread, per oz (28g)	175	1·1

Vegetables, Canned

	Calories	Fibre g
Artichoke hearts		
Wardour Artichoke Hearts, 14oz (400g)	115	2·5
Baked beans with tomato sauce		
Armour Baked Beans with Tomato Sauce, 7¾oz (220g)	140	16·0
Chef Baked Beans with 4 Pork Sausages, 7¾oz (220g)	270	13·5
Crosse & Blackwell Baked Beans with Tomato Sauce, 15½oz (439g)	280	32·0
Heinz		
Baked Beans with Tomato Sauce, 5·29oz (150g)	110	11·0

	Calories	Fibre g
Baked Beans with Tomato Sauce, 7·9oz (225g)	160	16·5
Baked Beans with Tomato Sauce, 15·9oz (450g)	325	33·5
Baked Beans with Pork Sausages, 7·9oz (225g)	285	11·5
Curried Beans with Sultanas, 7·9oz (225g)	195	16·5
S & W Barbecue Beans Chuckwagon Style in Tomato Sauce, 15½oz (439g)	315	33·0
Safeway		
Baked Beans with Tomato Sauce, 7¾oz (220g)	140	16·0
Baked Beans with Tomato Sauce, 15¾oz (447g)	285	32·5
Sainsbury's		
Baked Beans with Tomato Sauce, 7¾oz (220g)	155	16·0
Baked Beans and Sausages, 7¾oz (220g)	340	12·0
Tesco Baked Beans, 15oz (425g)	270	31·0
Waitrose Baked Beans, 5½oz (156g)	100	11·5
Barlotti beans		
Vulcano Barlotti Beans, 15oz (425g)	215	17·0
Broad beans		
Hartley's Broad Beans, 10oz (283g)	100	7·5
Smedley Broad Beans, 10oz (283g)	90	7·5
Waitrose Broad Beans, 10oz (283g)	120	10·5
Butter beans		
Batchelor's Butter Beans, 7½oz (213g)	115	6·5
Hartley's Butter Beans, 10oz (283g)	175	8·5
Safeway Butter Beans, 7½oz (213g)	115	6·5
Sainsbury's Butter Beans, 7¾oz (220g)	125	6·5
Tesco Butter Beans, 7½oz (213g)	125	7·0

	Calories	*Fibre g*
Cannellini beans (white kidney beans)		
Batchelor's Cannellini Beans,		
7·9oz (223g)	125	10·0
Bonduelle White Kidney Beans in		
Tomato Sauce, 14½oz (411g)	295	20·0
Vulcano White Kidney (Cannellini),		
15oz (425g)	240	18·5
Green beans		
Bonduelle		
Golden, Cut, 7¼oz (205g)	25	4·5
Whole Green Beans, 14½oz (411g)	20	9·5
Heley Cut Green Beans, 14½oz (411g)	50	7·5
Safeway		
Sliced Green Beans, 9½oz (269g)	20	3·5
Whole Green Beans, 14oz (397g)	15	7·0
Sainsbury's		
Cut Green Beans, 10oz (283g)	30	5·5
Cut Stringless Green Beans,		
14oz (397g)	40	7·5
Smedley Cut Green Beans, 10oz (283g)	15	5·0
Talpe Cut Green Beans, 14oz (397g)	35	6·5
Tesco Cut Green Beans, 10oz (283g)	30	5·5
Lima beans		
S & W Lima Beans, 16oz (454g)	310	26·5
Red kidney beans		
Batchelor's Red Kidney Beans,		
7·9oz (223g)	120	9·5
Pickerings Red Kidney Beans,		
15·9oz (450g)	240	19·0
S & W Red Kidney Beans, 8¾oz		
(248g)	130	11·5
Sainsbury's Red Kidney Beans,		
15½oz (439g)	230	19·0
Smedley Red Kidney Beans,		
10oz (283g)	260	20·0

	Calories	Fibre g
Stokeley Red Kidney Beans, 15oz (425g)	225	18·0
Tesco Red Kidney Beans, 15oz (425g)	285	19·5
Beetroot Baxter's		
Baby Beets, pickled, 12oz (340g)	155	8·5
Sliced Beets, pickled, 11¾oz (333g)	100	5·7
Brussels sprouts Bonduelle Brussels Sprouts, 14½oz (411g)	50	8·5
Talpe Continental Cuisine Brussels Sprouts, 14oz (397g)	45	7·5
Carrots Sainsbury's		
Sliced Carrots, 10½oz (298g)	35	6·5
Whole Carrots, 10½oz (298g)	30	6·5
Young Carrots, 7oz (198g)	25	4·5
Smedley		
Sliced Carrots, 10½oz (298g)	35	6·5
Whole Carrots, 10½oz (298g)	30	6·5

Mixed vegetables
Sainsbury's Mixed Vegetables
        (peas, carrots, turnips, potato),
    10½oz (298g)
	95	9·5

Smedley Mixed Vegetables
        (peas, swede, potato, carrot),
    10oz (283g)
	125	7·0

Tesco Mixed Vegetables
        (peas, carrots, potato, swede),
    10oz (283g)
	125	7·0

Mushrooms Chesswood		
Button Mushrooms in Brine, 7½oz (213g)	15	3·0

	Calories	Fibre g
Mushrooms (Chesswood), *cont.*		
Sliced Large Mushrooms in Brine, 7½oz (213g)	15	4·0
Sliced Mushrooms in Creamed Sauce, 7½oz (213g)	190	2·0
Small Whole Mushrooms in Brine, 7½oz (213g)	15	3·0
Sainsbury's Small Whole Mushrooms, 7½oz (213g)	15	3·5
Talpe Continental Cuisine Mushrooms, 7oz (198g)	15	3·0
Chick peas		
Bonduelle Chick Peas, 400g	275	14·5
Napolina Chick Peas, 15oz (425g)	275	14·5
Vulcano Chick Peas, 15oz (425g)	270	14·5
Garden peas and petit pois		
Bonduelle Petit Pois, 14½oz (411g)	125	13·5
Hartley's Garden Peas, 10oz (283g)	85	11·5
Safeway Petit Pois, 7oz (198g)	55	8·5
Sainsbury's		
Garden Peas, 5oz (142g)	45	6·5
Garden Peas, 10oz (283g)	90	13·0
Smedley		
Garden Peas, 5oz (142g)	60	4·5
Garden Peas, 10oz (283g)	125	9·5
Tesco		
Garden Peas, 10oz (283g)	85	13·0
Petit Pois, 10oz (283g)	90	13·0
Mushy peas		
Batchelor's Mushy Peas, 10·7oz (304g)	240	22·0
Sainsbury's Mushy Processed Peas, 10oz (283g)	220	23·0
Smedley Mushy Processed Peas, 10oz (283g)	240	9·0

	Calories	Fibre g
Tesco Mushy Processed Peas, 10oz (283g)	225	23·5
Peas pudding Pickering's		
Pease Pudding, 7½oz (213g)	290	11·0
Pease Pudding, 15oz (425g)	585	21·5
Sainsbury's		
Pease Pudding, 7¾oz (220g)	290	11·0
Pease Pudding, 15½oz (439g)	605	22·5
Processed and marrowfat peas Batchelor's Bigga Processed Peas, 10oz (283g)	150	15·0
Farrow's Giant Marrowfat Processed Peas, 4·97oz (141g)	70	6·5
International Processed Peas, 10oz (283g)	115	13·5

Safeway
    Marrowfat Processed Peas,
    10oz (283g)
	115	13·0

Processed Peas, 10oz (283g)	130	14·0
Sainsbury's Processed Peas, 10oz (283g)	130	14·0
Small Processed Peas, 10oz (283g)	145	14·5
Smedley Processed Peas, 10oz (283g)	190	10·5
Tesco Processed Peas, 10oz (283g)	140	15·5
Potatoes Sainsbury's New Potatoes, 10oz (283g)	115	5·5
Smedley New Potatoes, 10oz (283g)	135	3·5
Yeoman New Potatoes, mint flavour, 539g	190	9·0
Spinach Bonduelle		
Chopped Spinach, 7¼oz (205g)	55	11·5
Leaf Spinach, 14½oz (411g)	65	13·5

	Calories	*Fibre g*
Spinach, *cont.*		
Lockwood's Leaf Spinach, 9½oz (269g)	40	7·0
Smedley Spinach, chopped leaf,		
9oz (258g)	30	7·5
Talpe Chopped Spinach, 14oz (397g)	90	20·0
Sweetcorn		
Bonduelle Sweetcorn Kernels,		
12oz (340g)	220	16·5
Green Giant		
Mexicorn Golden Corn,		
whole kernels with peppers,		
7oz (198g)	150	10·5
Niblets Golden Corn, whole kernel,		
7oz (198g)	150	11·0
Kounty Kist Sweetcorn Kernels,		
12oz (340g)	200	17·5
Mexicana Sweetcorn with Peppers,		
11½oz (325g)	200	15·0
Sainsbury's		
Sweetcorn & Peppers, 12oz (340g)	230	17·5
Whole Kernel Sweetcorn, 7oz (198g)	150	11·5
Whole Kernel Sweetcorn,		
11½oz (326g)	250	18·5
Tesco Sweetcorn Kernels, 12oz (340g)	260	18·0
Tomatoes		
Mon Jardin Chopped Tomatoes,		
14oz (400g)	50	3·5
Napolina		
Peeled Plum Tomatoes, 8oz (227g)	25	2·0
Peeled Plum Tomatoes, 14oz (397g)	50	3·5
Regatta		
Italian Peeled Tomatoes, 8oz (227g)	25	2·0
Italian Peeled Tomatoes, 14oz (397g)	50	3·5
Sainsbury's Israeli Peeled Tomatoes,		
1lb 3oz (539g)	65	5·0

	Calories	Fibre g
Salads		
Bonduelle Mexican Salad		
(sweetcorn, peas, peppers),		
14½oz (411g)	165	15·5
Green Giant American Bean Salad,		
1lb 1oz (482g)	245	13·5
Heinz Vegetable Salad, 7¼oz (206g)	305	5·0

Vegetables, Dried

Whitworths		
Mixed Vegetables, per oz (28g) dry	75	7·0
Mushrooms, per oz (28g) dry	40	7·5
Peppers, per oz (28g) dry	60	3·5
Sliced Onion, per oz (28g) dry	85	4·5

Vegetables, Frozen

For basic frozen vegetables (e.g. peas) refer to Your Basic Calorie and Fibre Chart.

Stir-fry vegetables		
Birds Eye		
Continental Stir Fry Vegetables,		
10oz (284g), after frying	250	6·5
Country Style Stir Fry Vegetables,		
10oz (284g), after frying	250	6·5
Mediterranean Stir Fry Vegetables,		
10oz (284g), after frying	300	6·5
St Michael		
Brown Pack, 10oz (284g), as sold	90	6·0
Red Pack, 10oz (284g), as sold	80	10·0
Yellow Pack, 10oz (284g), as sold	130	8·0

Vegetable mixtures		
Birds Eye		
Casserole Vegetables, 8oz (227g)	80	5·5
Cauliflower, Peas and Carrots,		
8oz (227g)	80	9·5

	Calories	Fibre g
Vegetable mixtures (Birds Eye), *cont.*		
Original Mixed Vegetables, 4oz (113g)	60	5·5
Original Mixed Vegetables, 8oz (227g)	120	11·0
Peas, Sweetcorn and Peppers, 8oz (227g)	120	13·0
Rice, Peas and Mushrooms, 8oz (227g)	350	9·5
Rice, Sweetcorn and Peppers, 8oz (227g)	340	5·0
Ross		
Farmhouse Mixed Vegetables, 8oz (227g)	115	11·0
Mixed Vegetables, 8oz (227g)	125	12·5
Stewpack, 8oz (227g)	40	4·5

Wheatgerm

	Calories	Fibre g
Wheatgerm, per oz (28g)		
Allinson Wheatgerm (stabilized)	89	0·7
Bemax		
Crunchy	85	2·1
Natural Wheat Germ	85	2·1
Cheshire Wholefoods Wheatgerm	90	0·9
Froment Stabilised Wheatgerm	95	0·8
Granose Wheatgerm	102	2·0
Jordans Natural Wheatgerm	100	0·5
Kretschmer Wheatgerm (lightly toasted)	100	0·6

Drinks Calorie Guide

Drinks do not supply you with dietary fibre and do little, if anything, to satisfy the appetite – mostly passing through the stomach in a matter of minutes. That is why, in terms of weight control, it is generally better to eat a piece of fruit than to drink the juice.

There are many drinks, however, which are calorie-free and can be consumed with absolute freedom. These are listed on pages 61–62. Other drinks supply calories that must be included as part of your daily total.

Because alcoholic drinks lack nutritional value, those allowing themselves a little alcohol while following the F-Plan are recommended to have a minimum 1,000 calories (or 850 in the special circumstances described in Chapter 9) of food and drink, and add the alcohol-supplied calories to this total (see pages 63 and 64 for advice and instructions). There are very few people who would not achieve a speedy weight loss on a fibre-rich 1,200 calories a day, for instance, so you can ensure your nutrients by eating sufficient food and then allowing that little extra calorie ration for alcohol.

Many of the drinks listed here are not particularly recommended for F-Plan dieters; but they are included on the basis that if you are going to feel deprived without any one particular food or drink, it is better to include a little, while slimming, than to put too much strain on your will-power.

You will find an honest and realistic guide to alcohol calories here. We say 'honest' because a great deal of self-deception goes on in counting drinks calories during dieting. Pub measures can be relied upon for both meanness and accuracy. Home measures rarely can. It is so easy to count the calories for a single and then pour out very much more. And it is very dreary to have to measure precisely every tot or glass of wine.

For this reason, the number of calories in a whole bottle is often the safest and easiest guide to accuracy – and the most restraining influence – for home consumption. If you drink vodka, for instance, first decide how much to allow yourself for the week – perhaps a quarter or a half bottle. Then set that quantity aside in a separate bottle. Those are your alcoholic calories for the week, and when you've finished that's your lot – so an over-indulgent Monday could lead to a dry Saturday and Sunday. This way there is just no chance of making a multiplicity of little calorie mistakes with each drink, which could add up to many extra calories in a week.

With wines, the number of calories in a whole bottle tends to be the best guide, too. The size and fullness of different glasses of wine varies a great deal. Most people will either share a bottle of wine between two, with a meal, or perhaps share just half a bottle if they are dieting. Even from the sight of a glass of wine served in a restaurant or bar it is fairly easy to assess how many such glasses you would get from one bottle. Rather easier than thinking in terms of fluid ounces, for most of us!

So, in this chart, calories are given for full bottles as well as for full measures where applicable. There is a variation of about 50 calories between different bottles of wine in the groups we list together. For instance, sweet white wines will range from 600 to 650 calories. Unkindly, and to be on the safe side, we list the higher figure.

Drinks Calorie Chart

	Calories
Aperitifs, per bar measure	
Campari (50ml)	115
per bottle	1,840
Cinzano	
Bianco (50ml)	80
Rosso (50ml)	75
Dubonnet	
Dry (50ml)	55
per bottle	905
Red (50ml)	75
per bottle	1,255
Martini	
Bianco (50ml)	75
per bottle	1,255
Extra Dry (50ml)	55
per bottle	905

Beer, Cider and Lager, per $\frac{1}{2}$ pint (284ml)	
bitter	90
brown ale	85
cider	100
home-brewed beer	120
lager	90
light ale	75
mild ale	75
non-alcoholic lager (e.g. Barbican)	45
pale ale	90
special brew lager (e.g. Carlsberg Special Brew)	200

Beverages	
cocoa, 1 rounded teaspoon (10ml)	20
drinking chocolate, 1 rounded teaspoon (10ml)	20
Horlicks, malted milk, 1 rounded teaspoon (10ml)	20

	Calories
Beverages, *cont.*	
milk	
fresh, whole, pasteurized, sterilized, homogenized, longlife (UHT), or untreated farm milk, ½ pint (284ml)	180
fresh, semi-skimmed (e.g. Light Gold), ½ pint (284ml)	140
fresh, skimmed (e.g. Sainsbury's Vitapint Skimmed), ½ pint (284ml)	90
dried, skimmed, 1 rounded teaspoon (10ml)	10
Ovaltine, 1 heaped teaspoon (10ml)	25
tea, without milk, per cup	0

Fizzy Drinks and Mixers	
All 'low-calorie' labelled drinks (e.g. Energen One Cal Drinks, Diet Pepsi, Slimline Tonic) contain negligible calories	
American ginger ale, 4fl. oz (113ml)	40
Bitter lemon, 4fl. oz (113ml)	40
Coca Cola	
11½fl. oz (325ml) can	140
6½fl. oz (185ml) bottle	80
dry ginger ale, 4fl. oz (113ml)	40
lemonade, ¼ pint (142ml)	50
orangeade, 4fl. oz (113ml)	55
Pepsi Cola	
11½fl. oz (325ml) can	135
6fl. oz (170ml) bottle	70
Schweppes Slimline Shandy, 8½fl. oz (241ml) bottle	15
soda water, per glass	0
tonic water, 4fl. oz (113ml)	40

Fruit Juices, per 4fl. oz (113ml) glass	
apple	40
grape	60

	Calories
grapefruit	
bottled, sweetened	65
canned, unsweetened	35
canned, sweetened	45
in a carton (e.g. Just Juice)	25
frozen, reconstituted	45
orange	
bottled, sweetened	70
canned, unsweetened	35
canned, sweetened	55
in a carton (e.g. Just Juice)	40
frozen, reconstituted	60
pineapple	
canned, sweetened	65
bottled, sweetened	65
tomato, bottled or canned	25

	Calories
Fruit Squashes and Cordials, per fl. oz (28ml), undiluted	
blackcurrant	
cordial	30
health drinks (e.g. Ribena)	85
lemon	
barley water	30
squash or drink	30
lime juice cordial	25
orange squash or drink	35
whole grapefruit drink	30

	Calories
Liqueurs, per bar measure	
Benedictine (25ml)	90
Cointreau (25ml)	85
Crème de Menthe (25ml)	80
Drambuie (25ml)	85
Grand Marnier (25ml)	80
Kirsch (25ml)	50
Tia Maria (25ml)	75

	Calories
Port and Sherry	
sherry	
cream (50ml), small schooner	65
per bottle	1,100
dry (50ml), small schooner	55
per bottle	750
medium (50ml), small schooner	60
per bottle	820
port (50ml)	75
Spirits	
brandy, per bar measure (25ml)	50
gin, per bar measure (25ml)	50
rum, per bar measure (25ml)	50
vodka, per bar measure (25ml)	50
whisky, per bar measure (25ml)	50
brandy, gin, rum, vodka and whisky, per bottle	1,675
Wine	
red, per 4fl. oz (113ml) glass	
dry	80
sweet	95
rosé, per 4fl. oz (113ml) glass	80
white, per 4fl. oz (113ml) glass	
dry	75
sparkling	90
sweet	100

Your Basic Calorie and Fibre Chart

This is the chart to use for measuring and calculating various quantities of foods, and for adding up your own recipes and day's meals.

In this chart calorie and fibre values are given per oz (28g) of food. More precise fibre and calorie figures are given here (as opposed to rounded figures in the other charts, which suffice when dealing with larger total quantities).

Your Basic Calorie and Fibre Chart

Food	Calories per oz (28g)	Fibre g per oz (28g)
All Bran	70	7·9
Almond paste	124	1·8
Almonds, shelled, whole or ground	158	4·1
Apples		
eating, raw		
weighed with skin and core	10	0·6
flesh only	13	0·6
cooking		
raw, flesh only	10	0·7
baked or stewed without sugar	9	0·6
Apricots		
fresh		
raw, weighed with stones	7	0·5
stewed, without sugar, weighed with stones	6	0·4
dried		
raw	51	6·7
no-need-to-soak (e.g. Whitworths), raw	44	6·0
stewed without sugar	18	2·5
canned in syrup	30	0·4
Arrowroot	99	0·8
Artichokes, globe, boiled	4	0·3

Food	Calories per oz (28g)	Fibre g per oz (28g)
Asparagus, boiled	5	0·4
Aubergines, raw, flesh only	4	0·7
Avocado, flesh only	62	0·6
Bacon		
collar joint		
raw, lean and fat	89	0
boiled, lean and fat	91	0
lean only	53	0
gammon joint		
raw, lean and fat	66	0
boiled, lean and fat	75	0
boiled, lean only	47	0
gammon rashers		
grilled, lean and fat	64	0
grilled, lean only	48	0
back rashers		
raw, lean and fat	120	0
grilled, lean and fat	113	0
fried, lean and fat	130	0
middle rashers		
raw, lean and fat	119	0
grilled, lean and fat	116	0
fried, lean and fat	134	0
streaky rashers		
raw, lean and fat	116	0
grilled, lean and fat	118	0
fried, lean and fat	139	0
Baking powder	46	0
Bananas		
weighed with skin	13	0·6
flesh only	22	1·0

Food	Calories per oz (28g)	Fibre g per oz (28g)
Barcelona nuts, shelled	179	2·9
Barley, pearl		
raw	100	1·8
boiled	34	0·6
Bean sprouts		
raw	8	0·3
canned	3	0·8
boiled	10	0·3
Beans		
adzuki, dry weight	91	7·0
baked, canned in tomato sauce	18	2·0
black–eyed, dry weight	97	7·2
broad, boiled	13	1·2
butter		
dry weight	76	6·0
boiled	27	1·4
French, boiled	2	0·9
haricot		
dry weight	76	7·2
boiled	26	2·0
mung, dry weight	65	6·2
red kidney		
dry weight	76	7·0
boiled or canned drained	25	2·3
runner		
raw	7	0·8
boiled	5	1·0
soya		
dry weight	112	1·2
boiled	37	0·4
Beef		
beefburgers, frozen		
raw	74	0·1

Food	Calories per oz (28g)	Fibre g per oz (28g)
Bovril	49	0
Brain		
calf and lamb, raw	31	0
calf, boiled	43	0
lamb, boiled	35	0
Bran, wheat	58	12·3
Brawn	43	0
Brazil nuts, shelled	173	2·5
Bread		
brown	62	1·4
currant	70	0·5
Hi Bran	57	3·1
malt	69	1·4
soda, white	74	0·6
wheatgerm (e.g. Hovis, Vitbe)	64	1·3
white	65	0·8
wholemeal	60	2·4
Bread rolls		
brown		
crusty	81	1·7
soft	79	1·5
white		
crusty	81	0·9
soft	85	0·8
wholemeal (e.g. Allinson)	60	2·4
starch-reduced	108	0·6
Bread sauce	31	0·1
Breadcrumbs, white, dried	99	1·0
Broccoli tops		
raw	6	1·0
boiled	5	1·1

Food	Calories per oz (28g)	Fibre g per oz (28g)
Brussels sprouts		
raw	7	1·2
boiled	5	0·8
Buns, currant	85	0·5
Butter	207	0
Cabbage		
red, raw	6	1·0
savoy		
raw	7	0·9
boiled	3	0·7
spring, boiled	2	0·6
white, raw	6	0·8
winter		
raw	6	1·0
boiled	4	0·8
Cakes		
fruit		
plain	99	0·8
rich	93	1·0
rich, iced	99	1·0
madeira	110	0·4
sponge		
with fat	130	0·3
without fat	84	0·3
jam-filled	85	0·3
Carrots		
old		
raw	6	0·8
boiled	5	0·9
young, boiled	6	0·8
canned, drained	5	1·0

Food	Calories per oz (28g)	Fibre g per oz (28g)
Cashew nuts	157	4·0
Cauliflower		
raw	4	0·6
boiled	3	0·5
Celeriac, boiled	4	1·4
Celery		
raw	2	0·5
boiled	1	0·6
Cheese		
Baby Bel	80	0
Brie	88	0
Caerphilly	101	0
Camembert	84	0
Cheddar	115	0
cheese spread	79	0
Cheshire	95	0
cottage cheese	27	0
cream cheese	123	0
curd cheese	40	0
Danbo	98	0
Danish Blue	103	0
Double Gloucester	105	0
Edam	88	0
Emmenthal	115	0
Fetta	54	0
Gorgonzola	112	0
Gouda	100	0
Gruyère	115	0
Jarlsberg	95	0
Lancashire	109	0
Lymeswold	115	0
Mycella	110	0

Food	Calories per oz (28g)	Fibre g per oz (28g)
Parmesan	114	0
Philadelphia, soft cheese	90	0
processed, full fat	87	0
Quark		
less than 1% butter fat	22	0
less than 5% butter fat	33	0
less than 12% butter fat	47	0
Red Leicester	120	0
Roquefort	99	0
Sage Derby	112	0
skimmed-milk soft cheese	25	0
soft cheese, full fat	110	0
St Paulin	98	0
Stilton	130	0
Tome au Raisin	74	0
Wensleydale	115	0
Cherries		
eating, raw	11	0·4
cooking, raw	11	0·4
stewed without sugar, weighed with stones	9	0·3
glacé	59	0·4
Chestnuts, shelled	48	1·9
Chicken		
light meat only, raw	32	0
dark meat only, raw	35	0
light and dark meat mixed		
raw	34	0
no skin, boiled	51	0
no skin, roast	41	0
meat and skin, roast	60	0
Chicory, raw	3	0·4

Food	Calories per oz (28g)	Fibre g per oz (28g)
Chinese leaves	3	0·6
Chips, fried in deep fat	71	0·6
Chips (grill), frozen, grilled	40	0·6
Chips (oven), frozen, baked in oven	55	0·6
Chocolate drinking	102	0
milk	148	0
plain	147	0
Chocolates, fancy and filled	129	0
Choux pastry, cooked	92	0·4
Christmas pudding	85	0·6
Cockles, boiled, without shells	13	0
Cocoa powder	87	0
Coconut fresh	98	3·8
milk	6	0
desiccated	169	6·6
Cod fillets		
raw	21	0
boneless, baked	27	0
boneless, poached	26	0
boneless, steamed	23	0
fried in batter	56	0
frozen steaks, uncooked	19	0
steaks, fresh or frozen, grilled	27	0
smoked		
raw	22	0
poached	28	0

Food	Calories per oz (28g)	Fibre g per oz (28g)
Cod liver oil	252	0
Coffee		
ground, roasted, dry weight	80	0
instant powder or granules	28	0
Coffee and chicory essence	61	0
Coley		
raw	20	0
steamed, weighed with bones and skin	24	0
Condensed milk		
whole, sweetened	90	0
skimmed, sweetened	75	0
Corn oil	252	0
Corn-on-the-cob		
kernels only, raw	36	1·0
kernels only, boiled	34	1·3
Corned beef	61	0
Cornflakes	103	0·8
Cornflour	99	0·8
Courgettes		
raw	5	0·5
boiled	2	0·3
Cow's milk, fresh, whole	18	0
Crab		
boiled, meat only	36	0
canned	23	0
Cranberries, raw	4	1·2

Food	Calories per oz (28g)	Fibre g per oz (28g)
Cream		
double	125	0
half	35	0
single	59	0
soured	59	0
sterilized, canned	64	0
whipping	93	0
Crispbread		
rye	90	3·3
wheat, starch-reduced	109	1·4
Crisps, potato	149	3·2
Cucumber	3	0·1
Currants, dried	68	1·8
Custard		
egg	33	0
made with powder	33	0
Custard powder	99	0·8
Damsons		
raw	10	1·0
stewed without sugar	8	0·9
Dates		
dried		
no stones	69	2·4
weighed with stones	60	2·1
chopped and sugar-rolled	77	2·0
Dogfish (rock salmon), fried in batter	74	0·1
Dried milk, cow's		
whole	137	0
skimmed	99	0

Food	Calories per oz (28g)	Fibre g per oz (28g)
Dripping, beef	249	0
Duck		
raw, meat only	34	0
roast		
meat only	53	0
meat, fat and skin	95	0
Eel, stewed, flesh only	56	0
Egg		
whole, raw, without shell	41	0
boiled	41	0
fried	65	0
poached	43	0
Egg white, raw	10	0
Egg yolk, raw	95	0
Eggplant, *see* **Aubergines**		
Endive, raw	3	0·6
Evaporated milk, whole, unsweetened	44	0
Figs		
green, raw	11	0·7
dried		
raw	60	5·2
stewed without sugar	33	2·9
Fish fingers		
frozen	50	0·2
grilled without fat	50	0·2
fried	65	0·2
Flaky pastry, cooked	158	0·6

Food	Calories per oz (28g)	Fibre g per oz (28g)
Flour		
brown (85% extraction)	92	2·1
patent (40% extraction)	97	0·8
rye (100% extraction)	94	3·3
white		
bread-making (72% extraction)	94	0·8
household, plain	98	1·0
household, self-raising	94	1·0
wholemeal (100% extraction)	89	2·7
Frankfurters	77	0·3
Fruit gums	48	0
Fruit salad		
canned	27	0·3
dried, stewed without sugar	29	2·2
Gammon, *see under* **Bacon**		
Gelatine	95	0
Glacé cherries, *see under* **Cherries**		
Glucose, liquid	89	0
Goat's milk	20	0
Golden syrup	83	0
Goose, roast, meat only	89	0
Gooseberries		
green		
raw	5	0·9
stewed without sugar	4	0·8
ripe, raw	10	1·0
Grapefruit		
fresh		
weighed with skin and pips	3	0·1

Food	Calories per oz (28g)	Fibre g per oz (28g)
flesh only	6	0·2
canned in natural juice	11	0·1
canned in syrup	17	0·1
Grapefruit juice, canned		
unsweetened	9	0
sweetened	11	0
Grapenuts	99	2·0
Grapes		
black, raw	14	0·1
white (green), raw	17	0·3
Greengages		
raw, weighed with stones	12	0·7
stewed without sugar, weighed with stones	11	0·6
Groundnut (peanut) oil	252	0
Grouse, roast		
meat only	48	0
weighed with bone	32	0
Guavas, canned	17	1·0
Haddock fillets		
fresh		
raw	20	0
fried, weighed without bones	49	0
steamed, weighed without bones	27	0
smoked, steamed, weighed without bones	28	0
Halibut		
raw	26	0
steamed, flesh only	37	0

Food	Calories per oz (28g)	Fibre g per oz (28g)
Ham		
boiled, lean only	47	0
cooked and vacuum-packed	40	0
canned	33	0
Ham and pork, chopped, canned	76	0
Hare, stewed, weighed with bone	39	0
Hazelnuts, shelled	106	1·7
Heart		
lamb, raw	33	0
sheep, roast	66	0
ox		
raw	30	0
stewed	50	0
pig, raw	26	0
Herring		
raw, flesh only	66	0
coated in oatmeal, fried	66	0·4
grilled, flesh only	56	0
Honey, in jars	81	0
Horseradish, raw	17	2·3
Ice cream		
dairy	47	0
non-dairy	46	0
Jam		
fruit with edible seeds (e.g. raspberry)	73	0·3
stone fruit (e.g. plum)	73	0·3
Jelly		
packet cubes	73	0
made up with water	17	0

Food	Calories per oz (28g)	Fibre g per oz (28g)
Kidney		
lamb		
raw	25	0
fried	43	0
ox		
raw	24	0
stewed	48	0
pig		
raw	25	0
stewed	43	0
Kipper, baked		
flesh only	57	0
weighed with bones	31	0
Lady's fingers, *see* **Okra**		
Lamb		
breast		
raw, lean and fat, no bone	106	0
roast, lean and fat, no bone	115	0
roast, lean only	71	0
cutlets		
raw, lean and fat, weighed without bone	108	0
grilled, lean and fat, weighed without bone	104	0
grilled, lean and fat, weighed with bone	68	0
grilled, lean only	62	0
leg		
raw, lean and fat, weighed without bone	67	0
roast, lean and fat, weighed without bone	74	0

Food	Calories per oz (28g)	Fibre g per oz (28g)
Lamb, *cont.*		
roast, lean only	53	0
loin chops		
raw, lean and fat, weighed without bone	106	0
grilled, lean and fat, weighed without bone	99	0
grilled, lean and fat, weighed with bone	78	0
lean only	62	0
scrag and neck		
raw, lean and fat, weighed without bone	88	0
stewed, lean and fat, weighed without bone	82	0
stewed, lean only, weighed with fat and bone	71	0
shoulder		
raw, lean and fat, weighed without bone	88	0
roast, lean and fat, weighed without bone	88	0
roast, lean only	55	0
Lard	250	0
Laverbread (cooked, puréed seaweed, coated in oatmeal)	15	0·9
Leeks		
raw	9	0·9
boiled	7	1·0
Lemon curd		
starch base	79	0·1
home-made	81	0

Food	Calories per oz (28g)	Fibre g per oz (28g)
Lemon juice, fresh	2	0
Lemon sole		
raw	23	0
fried coated in crumbs, weighed with bones	48	0·1
steamed, weighed without bones	25	0
Lemons, whole, including skin	4	1·4
Lentils		
raw	85	3·3
split, boiled	28	1·0
Lettuce, raw	3	0·4
Liquorice Allsorts	88	0
Liver		
calf		
raw	43	0
fried	71	0
chicken		
raw	38	0
fried	54	0
lamb		
raw	50	0
fried	65	0
ox		
raw	46	0
stewed	55	0
Liver sausage	87	0·1
Loganberries		
raw	5	1·7
stewed without sugar	4	1·6
canned in syrup	28	0·9

Food	Calories per oz (28g)	Fibre g per oz (28g)
Milk, *cont.*		
dried		
whole, not made up	137	0
skimmed (e.g. Marvel), not made up	95	0
skimmed with added vegetable fat (e.g. Cadbury's Pint Size), not made up	140	0
skimmed with added vegetable fat, made up with water	14	0
cultured buttermilk	10	0
goat's milk	20	0
soya milk, diluted as instructed	18	0
Mincemeat	66	0·9
Minestrone soup, dried	83	1·8
Muesli	103	2·0
Mulberries, raw	10	0·5
Mushrooms		
raw	4	0·7
fried	59	1·1
Mussels		
raw, weighed without shells	18	0
boiled, weighed without shells	24	0
Mustard and cress, raw	3	1·0
Nectarines		
raw, flesh and skin, no stones	14	0·7
raw, whole fruit weighed with stone	13	0·6
Oatcakes	123	1·1

Food	Calories per oz (28g)	Fibre g per oz (28g)
Oatmeal, raw	112	2·0
Okra (Lady's fingers), raw	5	0·9
Olive oil	252	0
Olives, in brine		
weighed with stones	23	1·0
weighed without stones	29	1·2
Onions		
raw	6	0·4
boiled	4	0·4
fried	97	1·3
spring, raw	10	0·9
Orange juice		
fresh	11	0
canned		
unsweetened	9	0
sweetened	14	0
Oranges		
whole, weighed with peel and pips	7	0·4
flesh only	10	0·6
Ovaltine	106	0
Oxo cubes	64	0
Oxtail, stewed, weighed on the bone	26	0
Oysters, raw		
weighed with shell	2	0
weighed without shell	14	0
Papaya (pawpaw), canned	18	0·1
Parsley, raw	6	2·5

Food	Calories per oz (28g)	Fibre g per oz (28g)
Parsnips		
raw	14	1·1
boiled	16	0·7
Partridge, roast		
meat only	59	0
weighed on the bone	36	0
Passion fruit (Granadilla), raw, weighed with skin	4	1·9
Pastry, *see* **Choux pastry, Flaky pastry, Shortcrust pastry**		
Pawpaw, *see* **Papaya**		
Peaches		
fresh raw, flesh only	10	0·4
raw, weighed with stone	9	0·3
dried		
raw	59	4·0
stewed without sugar	22	1·5
canned	24	0·3
Peanut butter	174	2·1
Peanut oil	252	0
Peanuts		
fresh	160	2·3
roasted	160	2·3
Pearl barley, *see* **Barley, pearl**		
Pears		
eating		
flesh only	11	0·6
weighed with skin and core	8	0·5

Food	Calories per oz (28g)	Fibre g per oz (28g)
cooking		
raw, flesh only	10	0·8
stewed without sugar	8	0·7
canned	22	0·5
Peas		
fresh		
raw	19	1·5
boiled	15	1·5
frozen		
raw	15	2·2
boiled	11	2·2
canned		
garden	13	1·8
processed	22	2·2
dried		
raw	80	4·7
boiled	29	1·3
split, dried		
raw	87	3·3
boiled	33	1·4
chick		
raw	90	4·2
boiled	30	1·7
red pigeon, raw	84	4·2
Peppers, green		
raw	4	0·3
boiled	4	0·3
Peppermints	110	0
Pheasant, roast		
meat only	60	0
weighed with bone	38	0
Piccalilli	9	0·5

Food	Calories per oz (28g)	Fibre g per oz (28g)
Pickle, sweet	38	0·5
Pigeon, roast		
meat only	64	0
weighed with bone	28	0
Pilchards, canned in tomato sauce	35	0
Pineapple		
fresh, no skin and core	13	0·3
canned	22	0·3
Pineapple juice, canned	15	0
Plaice		
raw, flesh only	25	0
fried in batter	78	0·2
fried in crumbs	64	0·1
steamed, flesh only	26	0
Plantain		
green		
raw	31	1·6
boiled	34	1·8
ripe, fried	75	1·6
Plums		
Victoria dessert, raw, weighed with stones	10	0·6
cooking		
raw, weighed with stones	6	0·6
stewed without sugar, weighed with stones	7	0·6
Polony	79	0·2
Pomegranate pulp	22	0·3

Food	Calories per oz (28g)	Fibre g per oz (28g)
Pork		
belly rashers		
raw, lean and fat	107	0
grilled, lean and fat	111	0
chops		
loin, raw, lean and fat, weighed		
without bone	92	0
loin, grilled, lean and fat, weighed		
without bone	93	0
loin, grilled, lean and fat, weighed		
with bone	72	0
loin, grilled, lean only	63	0
loin, grilled, lean only, weighed with		
fat and bone	37	0
leg		
raw, lean and fat	75	0
roast, lean and fat	80	0
roast, lean only	52	0
Pork sausages		
raw	103	0·1
fried	89	0·1
grilled	89	0·1
Porridge (oatmeal made up with water)	12	0·2
Porridge oats	113	2·0
Potatoes		
old		
raw, peeled	24	0·6
boiled	22	0·3
mashed	33	0·3
baked, weighed with skin	24	0·7
baked, flesh only	29	0·7
roast	44	0·6

Food	Calories per oz (28g)	Fibre g per oz (28g)
Potatoes, *cont.*		
chip, medium-thick cut	71	0·6
new		
boiled	21	0·6
canned, drained	15	0·7
instant powder		
dry	89	4·6
made up	20	1·0
crisps	149	3·2
Prawns, boiled, shelled	30	0
Prunes		
dried		
raw, with stones	38	3·8
no-need-to-soak (e.g. Whitworths),		
raw	33	3·4
stewed without sugar	21	2·1
Puffed wheat	91	4·3
Pumpkins, raw	4	0·1
Quinces, raw, flesh only	7	1·8
Rabbit		
raw, meat only	35	0
stewed		
meat only	50	0
weighed on the bone	25	0
Radishes, raw	4	0·3
Raisins, dried	69	1·9
Raspberries		
raw	7	2·1

Food	Calories per oz (28g)	Fibre g per oz (28g)
stewed without sugar	7	2·2
canned in syrup	24	1·4
Ready Brek	109	2·1
Redcurrants		
raw	6	2·3
stewed without sugar	5	2·0
Rhubarb		
raw	2	0·7
stewed without sugar	2	0·7
stewed with sugar	13	0·6
Ribena, undiluted	64	0
Rice Krispies	104	1·3
Rice		
brown		
raw	100	1·2
boiled	36	0·4
white		
raw	103	0·7
boiled	34	0·2
Rice pudding		
home-made	37	0·1
canned	25	0·1
Rock salmon, fried in batter	74	0·1
Roe		
cod, hard		
raw	32	0
fried	57	0
herring, soft		
raw	22	0
fried	68	0

Food	Calories per oz (28g)	Fibre g per oz (28g)
Rosehip syrup, undiluted	65	0
Rye crispbread	90	3·3
Rye flour	94	3·3
Safflower seed oil	252	0
Sago, raw	99	0·8
Saithe (coley) raw	20	0
steamed, no bones	28	0
Salad cream	90	0
Salami	137	0
Salmon fresh, raw	51	0
steamed, flesh only	55	0
canned	43	0
smoked	40	0
Salsify, boiled	5	0·3
Sardines canned in oil		
fish only	61	0
fish plus oil	94	0
canned in tomato sauce	50	0
Sausages, see **Beef sausages, Pork sausages**		
Saveloy	73	0·1
Scallops, steamed, no shells	29	0
Scampi, in breadcrumbs, fried	88	0·3

Food	Calories per oz (28g)	Fibre g per oz (28g)
Scones, made from white flour	104	0·6
Scotch pancakes (drop scones)	79	0·4
Sea-kale, boiled	2	0·3
Semolina, raw	98	0·8
Semolina pudding	37	0·1
Shortbread, made from white flour	141	0·6
Shortcrust pastry made from white flour		
raw	127	0·6
cooked	148	0·7
made from wholemeal flour		
raw	119	1·6
cooked	140	1·9
Shredded wheat	91	3·4
Shrimps boiled, shelled	33	0
canned	26	0
Skate, fried in batter	56	0·1
Skimmed milk, cow's fresh	9	0
dried	99	0
Soda bread, *see under* **Bread**		
Sole, lemon, *see* **Lemon sole**		
Soya bean curd	21	0·3
Soya bean oil	252	0
Soya beans, yellow, dried	112	1·2

Food	Calories per oz (28g)	Fibre g per oz (28g)
Soya flour		
full fat	125	3·3
low fat	99	4·0
Spaghetti		
white		
raw	106	0·8
boiled	33	0·2
brown wholewheat		
raw	97	2·8
boiled	32	0·9
canned in tomato sauce	17	0·3
Special K	109	0·5
Spinach, boiled	8	1·8
Sprats, fried, whole fish	109	0
Spring greens, boiled	3	1·1
Sprouts, brussels, *see* **Brussels sprouts**		
Strawberries		
raw	7	0·6
canned in syrup	23	0·3
Suet		
block	251	0
shredded	231	0
Suet pudding, sweet, steamed	93	0·3
Sugar		
demerara	110	0
white (caster, granulated, icing)	110	0
soft brown	110	0
Sugar puffs	97	1·7

Food	Calories per oz (28g)	Fibre g per oz (28g)
Sultanas, dried	70	2·0
Sunflower seed oil	252	0
Sunflower seeds	137	1·0
Swedes raw	6	0·8
boiled	5	0·8
Sweetbread, lamb raw	37	0
fried, coated in egg and breadcrumbs	64	0·1
Sweetcorn raw, kernels only	36	1·0
boiled, kernels only	34	1·3
canned	21	1·6
Sweet potatoes raw, flesh only	25	0·7
boiled, flesh only	24	0·6
Syrup, golden	83	0
Tangerines flesh only, no peel or pips	10	0·5
weighed with peel and pips	6	0·4
Tapioca, raw	100	0·8
Toffees, mixed	120	0
Tomato chutney	43	0·5
Tomato juice, canned	4	0
Tomatoes raw	4	0·4
canned	3	0·3

Food	Calories per oz (28g)	Fibre g per oz (28g)
Tongue		
canned	60	0
lamb, raw	54	0
sheep, stewed	81	0
ox		
pickled, raw	61	0
pickled, boiled	82	0
Treacle, black	72	0
Tripe		
dressed	17	0
stewed	28	0
Trout, brown, steamed, weighed with bones	25	0
Tuna		
canned in brine	33	0
canned in oil	81	0
Turnip tops, boiled	3	1·1
Turnips		
raw, flesh only	6	0·8
boiled, flesh only	4	0·6
Turkey		
raw		
meat only	30	0
meat and skin	40	0
roast		
meat only	39	0
meat and skin	48	0
light meat	37	0
dark meat	41	0
UHT milk *see under* **Milk**		

Food	Calories per oz (28g)	Fibre g per oz (28g)
Veal		
cutlet, coated in egg and breadcrumbs, fried	60	0
fillet		
raw	31	0
roast	64	0
jellied, canned	35	0
Vegetable oils	252	0
Venison, roast, meat only	55	0
Vinegar	1	0
Walnuts, shelled	147	1·5
Watercress	4	0·9
Weetabix	95	3·6
Wheatgerm	100	0·6
Wheatgerm oil	252	0
Whelks, boiled, no shells	25	0
White pudding	126	1·0
White sauce		
savoury	42	0·1
sweet	48	0·1
Whitebait, whole fish, fried	147	0
Whitecurrants		
raw	7	1·9
stewed without sugar	6	1·6
Whiting		
fried, coated in crumbs, weighed with bones	48	0·1
steamed, weighed with bones	18	0

Food	Calories per oz (28g)	Fibre g per oz (28g)
Wholemeal bread, *see under* **Bread**		
Wholemeal flour, *see under* **Flour**		
Winkles, boiled, no shells	21	0
Yam		
raw, flesh only	37	1·1
boiled, flesh only	33	1·1
Yeast		
bakers', compressed	15	1·9
dried	47	6·1
Yogurt, low fat		
natural	15	0
flavoured	23	0
fruit	27	0
hazelnut	30	0·5
Yorkshire pudding	60	0·3